GREEK MEDICINE

ASPECTS OF GREEK AND ROMAN LIFE

General Editor: Professor H. H. Scullard

GREEK MEDICINE

E. D. Phillips

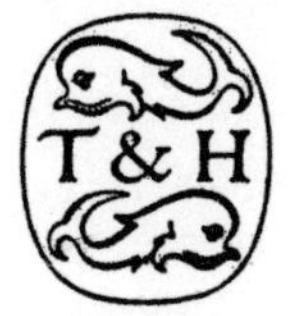

THAMES AND HUDSON

PRINTED IN GREAT BRITAIN BY
THE CAMELOT PRESS LTD, LONDON AND SOUTHAMPTON

ISBN 0 500 40021 0

CONTENTS

CONTENTS

LIST OF ILLUSTRATIONS

PREFACE

So far as I know, the present book is the first attempt made in English for many years to write an historical survey of Greek medicine. The account concludes with Galen both because of his great value as a source of information for earlier medicine and because after his time no important advances are known. Very little use has been made of general histories because most of these are antiquated; H. E. Sigerist's *History of Medicine* would have been an exception, but it was interrupted at an early stage by his death. As far as possible, every particular statement made rests directly on some piece of ancient evidence which will be found in the Notes. Editions of the Greek books have, of course, been used, and are listed in the Bibliography as well as being mentioned in the Notes.

The different aspects of Greek medicine are considered under the headings of modern medicine, so that the same ancient book is used several times over to answer different questions under modern headings. The questions are such as would occur to a modern reader who was interested in the actual achievements of Greek medicine, practical and theoretical. Some attention is given to questions of affinity and derivation, both among the medical writers and among the early scientists and philosophers, whose works are much more relevant than might be supposed.

The book is, therefore, addressed not only to Classical scholars who are interested in this department of Greek literature, and to their students, but also to historians of science and to all medical men who take a strong interest in the history of their profession. With this wider public in view, particular care has been taken not to place the medical science and practice of the Greeks on a higher level than the information warrants, but to show their pioneering efforts as they were, distinguishing between merely rational speculation and such hypotheses as could have been tested against observed facts.

These considerations have made it still more necessary to maintain everywhere the most concrete character that would be consistent with order and clarity. To achieve this concrete character, illustration is necessary, but this has raised another difficulty. The mass of detail in the Hippocratic Corpus alone is far greater than could be accommodated in a short historical summary, so that only a selection can be given. Any selection can be faulted as arbitrary by those who are familiar with Greek medicine; I have chosen what seemed to me interesting and important.

Thus in the Notes what may seem a disproportionate amount of reference is made to gynaecological matters. This is done partly because the subject-matter of gynaecology, beside its great importance in any system of medicine, happens to be concentrated on a small space within the female body, which is clearly marked off from surrounding organs and tissues and has a special character. Since some of it was easily observable for the physician and the midwife there are fairly full descriptions of its pathological states, even though some of the explanations of maladies are fantastic. The interaction of sound observation and sensible treatment with bizarre theory and interpretation illustrates well the merits and defects of Greek medicine.

The social history of medicine and the ethical attitudes of physicians among the Greeks are noted, with particular reference to those later periods from which most of our evidence on these subjects in fact comes. Much of this information is gathered into Chapter 9, 'The Medical Career'. My Appendix, 'The Cult of Asclepius', deals with an aspect of healing which must always be in the mind of any historian of Greek medicine even though the relation between faith-healing and rational medicine during these centuries is not easy to trace. I have tried throughout to avoid two faults of writing: excessive use of the technical vocabulary of medicine, which would be suitable neither for so early a stage of medicine nor for a lay author, and a literary manner which would only make a barrier between the reader and the subject treated. A general acknowledgment of help is due to various colleagues in the Faculty of Medicine at this University.

Belfast E. D. Phillips

CHAPTER I

INTRODUCTION

THIS BOOK IS AN ATTEMPT to survey the development of Greek medicine as practice and as science from the earliest mentions in extant literature down to the age of Galen, beyond whom there is little of scientific interest. The subject is a large one, and it has to be studied mainly in written texts. After the Hippocratic period of the fifth and early fourth centuries BC the texts are of very unequal value and interest, and some of the material, particularly such items as the accounts of drugs and their use, does not lend itself to convenient presentation in a general history or as a unified theory. The state of our later evidence is particularly unfortunate in that the writings of the Alexandrian anatomists and physiologists have perished, except for extracts, summaries and allusions preserved mainly in Galen. The corpus of Galen's own works, including his commentaries on the Hippocratic writings, is very large and miscellaneous in content, but he did frame a system of medicine which makes a fitting conclusion for our account.

Within the limits of the present book I have tried to present in brief summary with a little explanation and interpretation the entire spread of medical theory and information that is found in the so-called Hippocratic Corpus, but by no means always in the same order and context as is found in the separate books. Certain theoretical and polemical writings must be treated individually, like works of literature; but it has seemed to me much better, where strictly medical work is concerned, to extract much of the material from its setting in each book and to group it with corresponding material from other books under the categories of modern medicine. The loss of literary form required by this procedure may be regretted by Greek scholars, but for other readers, particularly if they are medically trained or are historians of science, this should be more than compensated for by the gain in intellectual order and clarity. They can thus judge what the Hippocratic contribution was under familiar headings.

Once the Hippocratic basis has been thoroughly described the works of later thinkers who added to it can be treated much more briefly. The Alexandrian school is important, but after that even the voluminous works of Galen are of less significance, except for their system of medicine already mentioned. Other writers will receive such mention as space allows, and something will be said of the various medical schools, some contemporary with the Coan school, to which Hippocrates belonged, and some later.

The history of Greek medical thought and practice is also an important part of the general history of science. Within the Greek achievement, medicine is second only to mathematics, and the Hippocratic writings have strong links with Ionian nature philosophy, which supplies many of their presuppositions even when they criticize it. In their own content they provide specimens of pre-Aristotelian biology which we should otherwise not possess, though they give no hint of the *scala naturae* which Democritus outlined in the same period as a forerunner of Aristotle. In physiology and anatomy the greatest progress known before the beginning of modern science was achieved by a few generations of physicians and surgeons working at Alexandria, where the Ptolemies allowed them to practise dissection and even some experimentation on living bodies. Galen's was the last thoroughgoing attempt to order the knowledge embodied in ancient Greek medicine.

As in other studies of Greek achievements, so here the question arises of borrowings made from the oriental civilizations which had a much longer experience of settled and civilized life. These borrowings occurred mostly in technique and in the knowledge of drugs. They are not the origin of Greek medical science as a persistent attempt to understand the workings of the living body and to build a coherent system of those workings. Nor does this science depend on the practice of temple medicine in the cult of

Asclepius, for the essence of this is faith-healing. Though temple medicine and medical science were not rival or hostile traditions among the Greeks, they were very much separate, in spite of the name Asclepiadae borne by the medical school of Cos. In our account the cult of Asclepius will be left on one side, despite the cures claimed for it and no doubt sometimes achieved, for it is not part of medical science.

Though the Greeks created rational medicine, their work was not always or even often fully scientific in the modern sense of the term. In the investigation of living things, for whatsoever purpose carried on, the complexity of empirical fact is so great that nothing of value can be established without constant observation, not to speak of experiment, to determine what is normal or healthy and what is abnormal or diseased. Like other Greek pioneers of science, the physicians were prone to think that much more can be discovered by mere reflection and argument than is in fact the case. Nevertheless this tendency, so strong in some of their writings, is in others continually criticized both on scientific and even more on practical grounds. For this reason also it is necessary at an early stage to relate the growth of medical science among the Greek physicians to the sweeping and curious judgments on the nature of things which are to be found in the remains of their contemporaries, the pre-Socratic nature philosophers. For in their time there was not yet a distinction, habitual with us, between philosophy and science, including medicine.

It was indeed no accident that scientific medicine among the Greeks began in the age of the nature philosophers, who swept away the magic and superstition that hindered its growth in other societies. But it was perhaps an accident that there was no powerful priesthood in Greece to cramp or block the advance of either form of thought.

Much of the traditional treatment for various injuries and ailments practised by the Greeks was inherited from folk medicine shared by them with other peoples. This would be natural for herbs and the more accessible drugs, of which the human race had collected knowledge piece by piece through the ages. Among well-known civilizations by whose medicine the Greek science was influenced, it appears that the Mesopotamian civilizations were not so important for theory in spite of their passion for listing diseases, and for numerical lore about disease.[1] The specialist healers who enjoyed great repute among them were in fact demonologists rather than doctors. But the Babylonians had good surgical instruments: scalpels, saws and trepans. Ordinary practitioners used traditional lists of treatments and remedies. With the Egyptians it is otherwise, for a well-defined profession of medicine with therapeutic, surgical, pharmacological and gynaecological skills existed from very early times, and the Greeks knew that this was so.[2] Perhaps the most important Egyptian notion found in papyri was that disease was due to putrefying residues of food carried in the bowels and giving off gases which permeated the body.[3] Hence the continual use of purges in Egypt, a practice which the Greeks followed. Among the Greeks these residues were called *περισσώματα*, 'superfluities', by the school of Cnidus.

The detail of these borrowings from oriental medicine is itself an interesting subject for research, but it cannot be pursued here; this is partly because of its complexity and obscurity, and partly because of the steady accumulation of new material from Egyptian papyri, Mesopotamian tablets and other sources. Very few scholars are able to understand these new finds properly, whether or not they compare them with Greek material.

From these general remarks on the nature and historical setting of Greek medicine we pass on to consider lay references to sickness, injuries and healing found in Greek literature down to the age of our medical texts proper, and in certain famous examples contemporary with those texts.

CHAPTER II

MEDICAL TOPICS AND CONCEPTIONS IN EARLIER LAY WRITERS

In Greek literature, as in most others, there are references of all kinds to health and disease, wounds and death, and to the agencies which cause them, whether natural or divine. Along with these references, which are mostly incidental, it will be convenient to include also doctrines or remarks found in the writings of the nature philosophers, where these have some physiological or medical content and are related to the thought of the medical writers themselves.

The earliest account of disease is the story in the *Iliad* of the plague sent by Apollo upon the Greek army before Troy in punishment for Agememnon's insulting the priest Chryses when he came to ransom his captured daughter.[4] Apollo begins to shoot his arrows, killing first the mules and dogs in the camp and then the Greeks themselves. This should be a mythical description of a disease with acute fever, sudden in onset and rapidly fatal, such as might easily attack an army. Nothing is said explicitly of any symptoms, nor even of any recoveries. However, when Apollo has been appeased with sacrifices and by the return of the girl, the Greeks set about cleansing the camp, throwing 'defilements' into the sea. This suggests that part of the disease was a severe dysentery leaving quantities of excrement, such as armies can suffer in the field. Apollo is addressed as *Smintheus* or 'mouser', which may be a sign that Homer saw mice as the source of infection. Rodents are indeed the original carriers of bubonic plague, acting as a reservoir of infection, and here the beginning of the infection among animals may be connected. But Homer has not written the medical report of an epidemic.

The arrows of Apollo and his sister Artemis, who shot at women, are often in myth a symbol for the sudden onset of disease, but they not only caused disease but could also heal it. In this capacity Apollo was called by the name of Paean, once a distinct god, whom he had absorbed into himself. He was also the father of the healer god Asclepius.

Asclepius had two sons who fought at Troy and also acted as healers, namely Machaon and Podalirius.[5] Machaon healed the wounds made by arrows, by drawing or, if necessary, cutting out the heads, washing the wounds, and sprinkling on them soothing remedies, the use of which he had been taught by the centaur Chiron.[6] They were perhaps powders made from dried herbs. Patroclus did the same with a 'bitter root' which had been shown him by Achilles, also a pupil of Chiron.[7] Warriors indeed treated one another without being professional physicians, but when Machaon himself was wounded in the right shoulder by a three-barbed arrow and treated in Nestor's tent, Idomeneus remarked: 'A healer is worth many other men for cutting out arrows and spreading gentle remedies upon the wound.'[8]

The practice of singing incantations (ἐπῳδαί) over wounds is not mentioned in the *Iliad*, but in the *Odyssey* Odysseus, wounded in his youth at a boar hunt, is said to have been bandaged skilfully by the sons of Autolycus, who stopped the bleeding with incantations.[9] Homer has many descriptions of wounds and injuries which show some knowledge of anatomy, but seldom mentions any treatment beyond washing and bandaging.

Though we do not possess the epic versions of heroic legends other than those treated by Homer, we have details which must descend from these. Thus in a scholium on Pindar's *Pythian Ode* I the treatment of Philoctetes' poisonous bite is described.[10] While he was asleep, Machaon cut away the gangrenous flesh from the festering ulcer, poured wine over it, and sprinkled on the wound a herb that Asclepius had obtained from Chiron. According to Quintus Smyrnaeus, Podalirius squeezed out wounds, stitched them up and spread on them salves that his father Asclepius had placed in his hands.[11] Podalirius indeed later came to be credited with skill in internal medicine in contrast to his brother's surgery. A scholium on *Iliad* XII quotes from Arctinus' *Sack of Troy*: 'For their father gave them both honours but made one more renowned than the other. To one he gave nimbler hands and the power of drawing missiles from the flesh and cutting it, and of curing all wounds; to the other the power of knowing accurately in his heart all unseen things and healing what could not be healed.'[12] In the poetry of heroic battle, detailed reference to internal illness was out of place, while full descriptions of wounding had a technical interest for the original audience of warriors. Yet the lines from Arctinus show the beginning of the distinction between medicine and surgery.

In Hesiod's *Works and Days* famine and plague are said to be sent by Zeus: men perish and women cease to bear children.[13] Hesiod notes that in winter a man in poverty who has not set aside food 'will press a thick foot with a thin hand'. General emaciation is represented in the hand, but the thick foot has been recognized as a case of nutritional oedema.[14]

Without entering on temple medicine, we find more detail of healing as understood by laymen in Pindar's *Pythian Ode* III, where Asclepius again figures. 'And whosoever came suffering from the sores of nature, with limbs wounded by grey bronze or far-hurled stone, or with bodies wasted by summer heat or winter cold, he delivered them, different ones from different pains, tending some with kindly incantations, giving some soothing potions to drink or fastening simples about their limbs, while he set some on their feet again with the knife.'[15] Such, according to Pindar, was the human medicine of Asclepius, when he still lived as a mortal on earth before being killed by Zeus and eventually becoming a god.

In Aeschylus' *Prometheus* the crazed figure of Io, wholly or partly changed into a heifer, is driven across the earth by the gadfly sent by Hera.[16] When the fit comes on, she is inflamed with *sphakelos* or gangrene about the sting and crazed by delirium, while her heart races, her eyes roll, and she cannot control her utterance. These are intended to be understood as the directly physical effects of the sting. In Cassandra's frenzied visions as shown in the *Agamemnon* there are similar features, but her wild utterance is prophecy rather than delirium.[17] In the *Eumenides* Aeschylus makes Apollo say that the mother has no share in begetting the child, but merely nurses the newly sown seed.[18]

In Sophocles' *Philoctetes* the snake-bite in the hero's foot makes him limp and cry aloud with the pain, while the flesh continually suppurates as the rodent ulcer spreads.[19] Philoctetes keeps a herb as a palliative, but the bleeding is renewed in every attack of pain. The frenzy that strikes Heracles in Euripides' *Mad Heracles*, or strikes the women of Thebes in *The Bacchae*, has a certain medical interest but is not treatable.[20]

More illuminating than these stray references are the historians. Herodotus tells how Cambyses, King of Persia, fell from his horse and was wounded when the chape came off the sheath of his sword and the point of the weapon pierced his thigh. The bone became gangrenous and the thigh putrefied.[21] No effective treatment is mentioned. The Greek physician Democedes of Croton won high favour at the Persian court after he was taken captive along with the household of Polycrates, tyrant of Samos, his profession being at first unknown. When King Darius dislocated his ankle out hunting, Egyptian physicians were first called in, whose violent methods caused such pain that Darius could not sleep for seven days and nights. Democedes on the other hand applied gentle methods which made it possible for the king to sleep; he recovered after giving up hope of ever again being sound in that foot. Darius rewarded Democedes and appointed him physician to his wives, in which capacity he cured a tumour on the breast of Atossa on condition that she helped him to return to Croton. He was thus sent on a Persian mission as far as Taras, whence he made his escape.[22]

A different interest attaches to Herodotus' remarks on the Egyptians' habit of purging themselves for three days every month. He says that they pursue health by purges and emetics and believe that all human disease arises from food. This practice, helped by the unchanging climate that they share with the Libyans, makes them the healthiest of mankind.[23] Herodotus' account is certainly confirmed by Egyptian sources, as we saw in Chapter 1.

A generation later Thucydides wrote his celebrated account of the plague at Athens.[24] This pestilence came from Ethiopia by way of Egypt during a year which had been otherwise free of disease. It began with hot headaches, redness and inflammation of the eyes, with bloodiness of the throat and tongue and peculiarly malodorous breath. Sneezing and hoarseness followed until the complaint descended to the chest, producing a violent cough. When it reached the entrance to the stomach it caused convulsion in it and every kind of evacuation of bile known to medicine. Empty retching came on, with violent spasms. The body was not too hot or cold to the touch, but it was reddish, livid, and covered in a rash of small pustules and ulcers. Sufferers could not bear the thinnest clothes. Many threw themselves into cold water suffering from unquenchable thirst, but much or little drink was the same to them. Their bodies did not waste at the height of the disease. Most of them died on the ninth or seventh day from internal burning, still keeping some of their strength; if they survived this, then when the disease descended to their intestines there followed violent ulceration with uniformly fluid diarrhoea, until most died of weakness. The disease went through the whole body from the head downwards, seizing eventually on the genitals, fingers, toes or eyes; some survived the loss of these. Those who recovered suffered from loss of memory. Birds and beasts in contact with men were also infected.

In spite of the apparently full description, generations of medical readers have disagreed with one another over the diagnosis. Suggestions have included bubonic plague and measles, but the most likely is considered to be typhus.[25] One point to be remembered is that any disease may have changed its symptoms somewhat over the centuries.

From these few literary references to purely medical matters we turn to the nature philosophers, whose remains are so fragmentary that their utterances seem more arbitrary and capricious than probably they were.

One of the most important is Alcmaeon of Croton,[26] a physician like his fellow-citizen Democedes, but a man of wider interests. He appears to have been the first to formulate the doctrine of health as a balance among the powers of the body, these powers being constituent fluids with definite qualities and causal properties. Health was ἰσονομίη, 'equality before the law', among these fluids, and illness μοναρχιή, the dominance of one of them. This conception was taken from the observed struggle of factions in politics. Among the indefinitely many qualities that needed to be held in balance were heat and cold, moisture and dryness, bitterness and sweetness; such qualities were permanently inherent in the fluids, which are the humours of Hippocratic medicine in an early stage.

Alcmaeon insisted on the difference between man and the lower animals, saying that man alone had understanding, the other animals only sensation. He taught that the brain was the seat of intelligence and that the sense organs were connected to it.[27] The ears transmitted sound because they contained void which resounded in the inner ear: void being, in his opinion, air. A man smelled with his nostrils as he drew breath up to the brain. Tastes were distinguished by the warm and soft tongue, which melted substances with its heat and, being porous and delicate, received and transmitted the flavours. The eyes saw through the water surrounding them and evidently contained fire, which flashed forth when they were struck; they saw by means of the bright element, and of the transparent one when that gave back a reflection. Since all the senses were connected to the brain, they were incapacitated if it was disturbed or shifted so as to block the transmitting passages.[28] Strangely enough, Alcmaeon has nothing to say of touch in extant fragments.

Though he could recognize or infer sensory channels, which he would have conceived as hollow vessels, Alcmaeon never recognized nervous tissue any more than his successors did before Alexandrian times. In physiology he held that sleep was caused by the retirement of the blood into the larger vessels, while waking resulted from its rediffusion. Among the parts left bloodless he no doubt included the brain.[29] He practised dissection to the extent of cutting out an eye, apparently from a living animal, but he is most unlikely to have done any dissection of human bodies.[30] He had a distinctive doctrine of the soul: that its immortality followed from its resemblance to the heavenly bodies which moved continuously and for ever. He argued that men die because 'they cannot join the beginning to the end', that is, cannot maintain continuous circulation of the 'soul-stuff' from the brain about the body and back again. The soul then left the body and death ensued.[31] Alcmaeon may be counted the remote founder of neurology.

No less important was Empedocles of Acragas in Sicily, who among other activities also practised medicine.[32] In his cosmological system the spherical universe was alternately dominated by Love, which mingled all the different elements, earth and fire and water, into a unified mass, and by Strife, which separated them into mutually exclusive layers. Living creatures appeared when each of these processes had gone halfway. Parts of them were formed before the wholes, and combined their ingredients in different ratios. Love and Strife were cosmic forces having a life of their own, as had the elements.[33]

In human growth male embryos are formed from the seed of both parents on the right side of the womb, which is hotter, and female ones on the left. As the embryo grows, tissues of each kind seize matter of their own kind for increase. In the growth of mules two soft stuffs combine in a hard dense mixture, as tin and copper combine to form bronze; they are thus infertile because the females are impermeable and cannot conceive. Echoes of this opinion are found later in the Hippocratics and in Aristotle. By means of the material presented to it in these elements, the intelligence of a man grows; he thinks, and feels pleasure and pain. We are aware of Love and Strife and of the elements by being composed of the same things ourselves. This may be called a doctrine of perception by chemical affinity; it is in contrast to the doctrine of Anaxagoras, to be mentioned later.

Empedocles had a special interest in respiration. He compared inspiration and expiration to the action of a water-lifter, *κλεψύδρα*, a vessel having a flat bottom pierced with holes and curving upwards hemispherically to a round mouth which could be stopped with the hand. A girl drawing water with this vessel pushes it down into the water, which rushes up through the holes. Then she closes the mouth with her finger and lifts out the water, which is kept by the air from running out through the holes until she opens the top again. So in respiration the air is drawn through fine holes in the inner surface of the nostrils as blood retires from them, and is driven out again when the blood returns in the regular oscillation of breathing; the blood in the body corresponds to the water in the vessel. This process works because blood-vessels contain some blood, but are not full of it, so that air can be present. The blood-vessels also have pores leading to the outer air, which are too small to let particles pass out from the body, but large enough to let in air.[34] This notion need not have been confined to the nostrils. Empedocles also taught that the blood about the heart was the organ of thought.[35]

In a remarkable fragment Empedocles claims to be able to reveal remedies for all disease and a way of warding off old age, how to stop the winds and call them up again, how to make seasonable drought after rain, how to bring seasonable streams to nourish the trees after drought, and even how to restore a dead man to life.[36] These claims show that though he could think of medical and biological matters in a rational way he did not cease to be a prophet and a wizard. He is also said to have saved the people of Selinus from disease caused by a stinking river by diverting two other rivers into it, a feat which could be called one of sanitary engineering.[37]

Contemporary with Empedocles was Anaxagoras of Clazomenae in Ionia, whose cosmological theory has an important bearing on his view of physiology, particularly of nutrition.[38] The relevant part of his doctrine concerned the constitution of matter.[39] In his view, every piece of matter, regardless of its size or kind, contained within it not only parts of the character that dominated the whole of it, but also parts having every other of the infinitely many characters found in the stuff of the universe. Furthermore, matter was, not only in geometrical theory but in fact, infinitely divisible. Thus, when any amount of matter changed its character, or when matter of a new character seemed to appear, this was in fact no more than appearance, since the new character had formerly been latent while another was dominant, and now merely became dominant itself. In this way change occurred without making anything appear out of nothing. In physiology, where perhaps Anaxagoras first conceived it, the theory explained nutrition: how, out of bread or other foods unlike the tissues of the body, these tissues could none the less be built up or replenished.

This doctrine, which assumed processes below the level of perceptible magnitude, was not capable of empirical proof; but the difficulties with which it was intended to deal are real enough. They have been solved in modern chemistry by a theory of particles of varying size and complexity. Each of these is a fairly stable structure of smaller particles but can in definite circumstances be replaced by another structure of the same smaller particles with some additions or losses, which presents a different appearance to sense. The infinite divisibility of Anaxagoras is replaced by a definite stop at each layer beyond which division can be continued only on different terms. Although Anaxagoras' theory was part of the background for the Hippocratic writings, it is not easily traceable in them. However, his claim that sensation arises by differences between the bodily sense organs and perceived things, not by affinity, did have some applications.[40] Assimilation, when it occurred, would be the end of perception.

Anaxagoras also held, like Alcmaeon, that the head and not the heart was the central organ of perception and thought, that it was the first part of the embryo to be formed and that the male alone produces seed in reproduction.[41] In the last of these opinions he agrees with Aeschylus, as we have seen.

Closer than Anaxagoras to the medical writers, who can be seen to use his ideas, was Diogenes of Apollonia.[42] Like one earlier nature philosopher, Anaximenes, he believed that all things were modifications of one substance, air or *pneuma*. Air is the universal stuff, but it is most active not in its modified states, where it appears as the other elements, but in its original one; for it is not only alive but intelligent and divine, and the cause of order in nature, evidenced by such things as the succession of the seasons. For animals and men who breathe it, it is soul and mind; it is great, strong, eternal and immortal, knowing many things, in fact God. The air in living bodies, which is consciousness, is warmer than most air outside, and must be kept dry lest it lose its power of thought. Men are able to keep it drier than other animals, which eat moister food and keep their heads closer to the earth. Air when breathed in is first massed in the brain and then carried along with blood about the body. Abundant air makes pleasure; lack of it, sluggish blood and pain; complete loss of it, death. It is active in semen, while the female contributes nothing to reproduction. The absurdities of this doctrine are apparent even in this bare recital; Aristophanes, who knew it well, makes fun of it in the *Clouds*.[43] Yet it is at least a strong influence in several of the Hippocratic books.

In detailed physiology we have Diogenes' account of the vascular system as preserved by Aristotle.[44] There are two great vessels running through the whole cavity of the body on either side of the spinal column, downwards to the legs and upwards under the collar-bone through the neck to the brain. From each of these, smaller ramifying vessels run off to all parts on its own side of the body, including two to the heart. Of the great vessels, the one on the left, the *splenitis*, communicates with the spleen, left kidney and left leg; the other, the *hepatitis*, communicates with the liver, right kidney and right leg. A pair of vessels called *spermatitis* run from the kidneys to the testicles or womb according to sex. In this system the brain was the principal organ, and its attachment to the two main vessels of the body is specially indicated, while the heart is mentioned only incidentally. The idea of two great veins, symmetrical with one another and identical in function, must be based on some observation of the aorta and the *vena cava*, probably in animals. In the fragment nothing explicit is said of the lungs or of anything like the pulmonary circulation. Veins are not distinguished from arteries, nor were they by nearly all the Hippocratics. By carrying vital air they function as the nervous system does in more developed anatomy and physiology to account for sensation and movement. In the genitals this blood becomes exceptionally warm and frothy with *pneuma*.

A system like that of Diogenes but more uncouth is outlined in the Hippocratic fragment *The Nature of Bones*, so called from its opening words, and in Aristotle's *History of Animals*, where it is attributed to Syennesis, a pupil of Hippocrates.[45]

A distinguished figure, who may close this series, is Democritus, who anticipated Aristotle in the range of his interests, including medicine and physiology.[46] His general theory of indestructible atoms in perpetual motion is not an influence in the Hippocratic writings, as it is in some later medical theory, but others of his doctrines are relevant to them. He held that the soul was composed of specially light and smooth atoms, like those of fire, though not identical. The special location of soul-atoms was in the head, but they travelled through the body to give it life. They were always attempting to leave the body under pressure from the atoms outside it, but since the air contained many other soul-atoms these were introduced in respiration to replace them. When the pressure from outside grew too great respiration ceased and death followed as the soul flowed out. Sleep was the same outflow in milder form. Sensations were effects of outer bodies and their atoms on the sense organs and varied with the state of the sense organs. These ideas of 'soul-stuff' could be expressed without atomism.

In biology the most relevant of his opinions concern reproduction and embryology.[47] In his view *pneuma* or vital air composed of soul-atoms is the vehicle of life and occurs in the semen too. It is collected from every part of the body, as was commonly supposed in ancient medical theory. Both parents contribute seed, according to Democritus, who agrees here with Alcmaeon and Empedocles. The sex of the embryo is determined by the preponderance of male or female seed, as in Alcmaeon. The first part to be formed is the umbilical cord, which provides an anchorage for it as it grows. The outer parts, such as head and belly, take shape before the inner. The embryo feeds itself by sucking cotyledons, structures like nipples set in the lining of the womb. Cold dilates the foetus, so that miscarriage is commoner in warm climates where this does not happen.

Democritus also wrote lost works on medical instruction, on regimen, and on prognosis. He is known to have treated breathing as most important and to have described the healthy condition of the eye and ear. He taught that excessive heat or cold impaired the power of thought.

These speculations and doctrines of the nature philosophers served as a necessary background for the theoretical side of

Hippocratic medicine; medical writers chose from among them what seemed suitable. Thus nature philosophy was for the Hippocratics and others what general science is for modern medicine.

CHAPTER III

THE BEGINNINGS OF PROFESSIONAL MEDICINE AND THE HIPPOCRATIC CORPUS

WE HAVE NOW REACHED the borders of professional medicine as it was understood by the Greeks. At some time between the age of Hesiod and that of the pre-Socratic nature philosophers, and before the use of a special kind of prose for medical writings, the medical profession developed in Greece. We can see that its origins were practical, but we cannot trace them directly before the fifth century.

Some notion of earlier tradition can be gained from the Hippocratic book *Ancient Medicine* (or *Sound Tradition in Medicine*) which was written about the middle of the fifth century by a physician devoted to traditional lore and technique, though familiar with contemporary theory.[48] He attacks the hypotheses or crudely simplified explanations of the nature philosophers and defends an existing craft of proved worth, which, in trying to preserve human life and health, has been forced to recognize the complexity of fact. Medicine for him is mainly a matter of regimen, particularly of diet, discovered by man under stress of necessity and continually improved. It has contributed much to the advance of man from a brutish condition in which he lived insecurely on strong and indigestible foods to a state of civilization in which cooking was one of the necessary arts. The author evidently sees medicine in this wide sense, which would include folk medicine, as an art both practical and intellectual, which is necessary to achievement of full humanity, and of which a profession has rightly been made. This art he regards as having developed through centuries of experience.

A natural method, and the favourite one in antiquity, of ordering and presenting the further history of Greek medicine is to treat it as the interaction of named medical schools. It is presupposed in such expressions as *Coan Prognoses* and *Cnidian Opinions*, which are found in the Hippocratic Corpus and recall the classification of philosophical schools from Plato's time onwards.[49] But in dealing with the Hippocratic writings themselves, traditionally attributed to Hippocrates of Cos, we find a great variety of interest and treatment, if not outright contradiction, so that they cannot all be used as evidence for the views of one medical school. Physicians of the various schools knew and used the work of other schools in a spirit of honourable rivalry, not of intolerance, so that fundamental notions of anatomy and physiology, as we should call them, run right through various writings with little modification. In the earlier days of Greek medicine the schools represented local traditions rather than opposite opinions, and did not resent one another as enemies or heretics. Only later did medical sects arise which did behave in this way.

In the tradition reported long after the Classical period by Galen in his *Method of Healing*, the greatest prominence among early physicians is given to the Asclepiad guild, found on the island of Cos and in the town of Cnidus facing it on the mainland of Asia Minor.[50] The Asclepiadae were no doubt in origin a family that had increased in number, particularly by accepting those who married into it. Those of Cos came to form a separate school from those at Cnidus. Of other schools the most renowned was that of southern Italy represented by Empedocles, Philistion, Pausanias and their friends.[51] Galen says that the Coan school was the best and the largest, but that the other two were not far behind it.[52]

Hippocrates, the second and the most famous physician of that name, is reported to have been the leader of the Coan school of physicians.[53] A genealogy of him was given in tradition, but no doctrine of the school is known before his time. His doctrine is very slightly attested in our earliest sources, but by Galen's time he had come to be regarded as the author of most of the Hippocratic Corpus, as it is now called. The growth of this opinion will be discussed later: first we have to notice the testimony of Plato and of the Aristotelian school.

In a well-known passage of the *Phaedrus* Plato shows Socrates comparing medicine, as knowledge of the body, with rhetoric, the art of persuasion, as knowledge of the soul, and asking whether the nature of the soul can be determined without knowledge of 'the whole'.[54] Phaedrus answers that according to Hippocrates and true doctrine it is impossible without this method to know the body either. We must first ask whether it is a simple or a complex thing; if simple, we must determine what power it has of affecting another thing or being affected by it, and if it has many elements we must enumerate these, and then see, as with the simple object, how each can affect anything or how it can be affected by it. Without this procedure there is no scientific knowledge.

There has been much argument over the meaning of 'the whole'. Some interpreters take it as 'the universe', particularly as understood by the nature philosophers;[55] others, with more show of reason, as 'the whole of the thing in question', and so, in medicine, the general physiology of the body.[56] Celsus remarks that Hippocrates of Cos was the first to distinguish medicine from philosophy.[57] If he had in mind the doctrine of *Ancient Medicine*, among the writings that were reckoned as Hippocratic, that would suit this passage of Plato, provided that 'the whole' meant 'the whole body'.

The other testimony is in the papyrus known as *Anonymus Londinensis*, dated to the second century AD and full of gaps, of which part consists of an account of early medicine with the quoted views of well-known physicians.[58] The anonymous writer credits his information on early medicine to Aristotle, but modern scholars, relying on a passage of Galen, attribute it to Aristotle's pupil Menon, who was set to compile a history of medicine, and they argue that our author depends on Menon's history at several removes. Thus the substance of his account would go back to the time of Aristotle.[59]

According to Menon, Hippocrates attributed diseases to the residues of too varied or too strong and indigestible foods which cannot be mastered.[60] The residues arise from their incompatible natures, and from them gases (φῦσαι) arise which bring on diseases. Hippocrates adopted this view because he held that breath (here πνεῦμα) is the most necessary component in our bodies, which when it passes about freely produces health and when it is impeded, disease. We are like the plants called 'soldiers': as they are rooted in moisture, so we are rooted in air by our nostrils and by our whole body. As the 'soldier' plants move from one piece of moisture to another, so we change our position in the air. The air that we breathe in is our supreme component.[61] On this theory when residues occur they give rise to breaths (φῦσαι) which, rising as vapour, cause diseases, and do so particularly by their changes, which determine the nature of the disease.

This is Aristotle's view of Hippocrates, says the papyrus, but Hippocrates himself says that diseases are caused by the differences in the elemental components of the human organism. These diseases arise through inflammation from the chilling and heating of bile. Hippocrates goes on to say that diseases have their origin in the air or in regimen. When the air produces a disease, it will be the same for all, but many different forms of disease occurring at the same time are due to individual errors of regimen. This last argument the writer claims to be unsound.[62]

Our papyrus cannot derive all its information from Aristotle or Menon, for it is inconsistent with itself and leaves a confused impression. The theory of residues producing gases (φῦσαι), which are the origin of disease, is quite different from the doctrine of bodily components and inbreathed air (πνεῦμα) as the cause of disease. Both types of theory are represented in the Hippocratic Corpus, the one for instance in *Diseases* I, the other in *Airs, Waters, Places*, but they are hardly compatible, at least as explanations of the same diseases.[63] The late writer of the papyrus was surely capable of confusing different doctrines precisely because there is such a variety in the Corpus, which by his time, the second century AD, was nearly all attributed to Hippocrates. For him anything reported by Menon of Hippocrates would need to be squared with anything found in the miscellaneous Corpus. For us the Corpus is a collection of writings illustrating a variety of medical traditions.

It is not easy to relate the testimony of Plato to the confused account given by the papyrus. But at least the theory of residues and gases seems too limited to account for disease of the whole body, while the doctrine of harmony among the elemental components and of the general effects of πνεῦμα could be regarded as the content of the doctrine of 'the whole', if the whole is in fact the organic body.

Using the passage from the *Phaedrus* and the reported doctrine of harmonious components and πνεῦμα, some scholars have attempted to define further the doctrine of Hippocrates and his Coan pupils as illustrated in some books of the Corpus. They have called it 'meteorological medicine', applied to all the organs of the body.[64] Certainly the tendency of books recognized as Coan is to give a general account of illnesses, using clinical experience and attempting not distinctive diagnosis, but a useful prognosis of the course of any illness. In that early state of medicine this unscientific procedure was probably of more use than refined differentiation.

The Cnidian school was of equal antiquity with the Coan.[65] The Cnidians are said by Galen to have delighted in distinguishing varieties of disease in each organ; seven in the gall-bladder, twelve in the urinary bladder, four in the kidneys, two in the thigh, five in the foot, four kinds of stranguria, three of phthisis, many varieties of quinsy and many diseases of the entrails.[66] According to Galen some of the school were criticized by Hippocrates for being ignorant of the specific and generic differentiae of diseases, which, as stated, is an Aristotelian rather than a Hippocratic stricture.[67] This attempt to catalogue varieties for sheer love of classification was a trait of the Greek intellect at most times, as can be seen from Plato's *Sophist* and from comedy, not to speak of Aristotle. It is a sound scientific procedure but only when information is abundant enough to make precise differentiation useful and important, as when the diseases may be superficially and initially alike but show different natures later.

The best-known physician of this school, and its founder, was Euryphon, of whom Menon says that he attributed diseases to nutriments not discharged by the belly but left as residues which then rise to the regions about the head.[68] Galen says that the lost

Cnidian Opinions was attributed to him, and that he was the author of some works attributed to Hippocrates; also that he was skilled in anatomy, wrote much on remedies, and particularly on human milk from the breast for consumptives.[69]

The Cnidian approach to disease is clearly indebted to the Egyptian. Some scholars suggest that Coan medicine by contrast draws on Mesopotamian tradition, but this seems hard to confirm. Cnidian doctrine appears in some pathological and gynaecological books of the Corpus.[70]

Menon mentions also a later Cnidian, Herodicus, who had a rather different doctrine of residues.[71] He held that nourishment taken without previous exercise is not assimilated, but lies in the belly undigested and unaltered until it turns to residues. The residues produce two liquids, an acid and a bitter, which have different effects according to their strength, their blending and the places where they occur, such as the head, the liver or the spleen. Herodicus is no doubt the gymnastic trainer of that name mentioned by Plato, who turned physician and became famous for over-exercising his patients even in fever.[72] Some books on regimen in the Corpus show traces of his attitude to diet.

Little is known of Italiote and Siceliote medicine in the fifth century, apart from Alcmaeon and Empedocles, who have already been treated in their medical aspects. For the fourth century we have their successor, Philistion of Locri, whom Plato knew and admired but who has left no works, though he is said to have written at length on diet.[73] According to Menon, Philistion thought that the human body was composed of the four traditional elements with their usual properties, as in Empedocles.[74] Disease he attributed to excess of heat or moisture, to sudden change from one to the other, to nourishment that was unsuitable or corrupted, and to wounds and sores. When breath passed through the whole body health resulted, for breathing is carried out not only by the mouth and nostrils but by the whole body. Where breath was hindered disease could also occur. In health, the breath cooled the innate heat which was centred on the heart but reached the lungs. The lungs took up not only air but also fluids.[75]

Philistion's doctrine has been traced in the Hippocratic book

The Heart, which is late.[76] He practised and taught in Syracuse early in the fourth century, and had as pupils the Cnidians Chrysippus the Elder and his disciple Eudoxus, who arrived from Egypt. His influence appears also in Diocles of Carystus. If we knew more of such relationships we should almost certainly find that the medical schools were not at all isolated from one another.

We pass now from these names and from the scraps of evidence for medical views associated with them to the great bulk of the Hippocratic Corpus, which by contrast has no authors' names for its treatises. There has naturally been constant debate about the authorship of the various books, at first directed at deciding at least what were the 'genuine works of Hippocrates'. This has led to no firm conclusions. The tentative deduction of one authority in a published lecture on this subject seem the most likely: that the books of the Corpus are the contents of a medical library belonging to the master physician of a school, who if he was the master, say, of the Coan school would welcome books from other schools such as the Cnidian.[77] The collection may have been named after Hippocrates because he was its collector and first owner. A copy of the collection, or even the original, could have been brought by pupils of Praxagoras of Cos to Alexandria, where it was preserved. Hippocrates may have written some or none of the books which we have.

In these circumstances it is useless to search for the style and personality of Hippocrates among the books, though many should contain his doctrine in some form. It is more useful to classify the books according to subject, doctrine, nature and purpose. This is an historical and to some extent a literary undertaking. Later it will be necessary to group them from a different point of view, according to their medical content as defined by the categories of modern medicine, in so far as these apply.

In Littré's complete edition (1839–61), which has ten volumes including the index, the books of the Corpus are printed with French rendering facing the Greek text in the following order: *Ancient Medicine* (I, 560–637), *Airs, Waters, Places* (II, 13–93), *Prognostic* (II, 94–191), *Regimen in Acute Diseases* (II, 224–77), with the spurious *Appendix* to it (II, 394–529), *Epidemics* I (II, 598–717), *Epidemics* III (III, 24–149), *Head Wounds* (III, 186–261),

In the Surgery (III, 272–337), *Fractures* (III, 414–563), *Joints* (IV, 79–327), *Leverage* (IV, 340–94), *Aphorisms* (IV, 458–609), the *Oath* (IV, 629–33), *Epidemics* II (V, 72–139), *Epidemics* IV (V, 144–259), *Epidemics* V (V, 208–59), *Epidemics* VI (V, 266–357), *Epidemics* VII (V, 364–469), *Humours* (V, 476–503), *Prorrhetic* (V, 511–73), *Coan Prognoses* (V, 588–732), *The Art* (VI, 3–27), *The Nature of Man* (VI, 33–69), *Regimen in Health* (VI, 72–87), *Breaths* (VI, 90–115), *The Use of Fluids* (VI, 118–37), *Diseases* I (VI, 142–205), *Affections* (VI, 208–72), *Places in Man* (VI, 277–349), *The Sacred Disease* (VI, 352–97), *Ulcers* (VI, 400–33), *Haemorrhoids* (VI, 436–44), *Fistulae* (VI, 449–61), *Regimen* II or *Dreams* (VI, 630–63), *Diseases* II and III (VII, 8–161), *Internal Affections* (VII, 166–303), *The Nature of Woman* (VII, 312–431), *The Seven Months' Child* and *The Eight Months' Child* (VII, 436–61), *Diseases* IV with *Seed* and *The Nature of Child* included in the ancient text (VII, 472–615), *Diseases of Women* I and II (VIII, 10–407), *Sterile Women* (VIII, 408–63), *Diseases of Girls* (VIII, 467–70), a fragment, *Superfoetation* (VIII, 477–509), *Excision of the Foetus* (VIII, 512–19), *Anatomy* (VIII, 539–41), *Teething* (VIII, 544–9), *Glands* (VIII, 556–75), *Fleshes* or *Tissues* (VIII, 584–615), *Sevens*, on the grouping of medical things and events in sevens, in Latin translation only (VIII, 634–73), *Prorrhetic* II (IX, 6–75), *The Heart* (IX, 80–93), *Nutrition* (IX, 98–121), *Vision* (IX, 152–61), *The Nature of Bones*, so called from its first words (IX, 163–97), *The Physician* (IX, 204–21), *Decorum* (IX, 226–45), *Precepts* (IX, 250–73), *Crises* (IX, 276–95), *Critical Days* (IX, 298–307), *Letters, Decree* and *Addresses*, fictitious, attributed to Hippocrates in public roles (IX, 312–429), further MS of *Sevens*, also in Latin (IX, 433–66).

From this list, which is reproduced from Littré without any consideration of later enquiries into the interrelation of the books, the range of the collection is obvious, if not the exact nature of each book. In the remainder of this chapter some of the provisional conclusions of later scholarship will be given on the grouping of the books according to doctrine and school. To attempt to date them closely is for the most part a foolish enterprise; all that can be said is that they appear to belong to the second half of the fifth century, with some continuation into the early fourth.

An attempt to build up a Coan group of writings within the Corpus has been made by some authorities, who take the 'whole' in the *Phaedrus* as meaning the universe.[78] They do this with the intention of ascribing books to Hippocrates himself, but, apart from Hippocrates, their work has its value in showing that one Coan doctrine – that of 'meteorological medicine' – and one attitude run through these books in spite of differences in purpose and interest.

Much more meaning is latent in the term 'meteorological' than might appear. It presupposes the general approach to nature, including living creatures, which is found with individual variations in the nature philosophers briefly mentioned in an earlier chapter. In that chapter obvious links were shown between recognizably medical interests appearing in some of the nature philosophers and the general subject matter of the Corpus. The important point is that for the nature philosophers μετεωρολογία, as it was called in a hostile and scornful tone late in the fifth century, included all the visible and invisible processes of change among the elements on and above the earth. The elements made up the physical environment of a man and had effects on him, particularly through his breathing, drinking and eating, by which he took them into his body. This certainly agrees well with the interpretation of the 'whole' as the universe, particularly as the simple universe of the Ionian cosmologists; but we are still not forced to believe that Hippocrates' 'whole' was the universe, for the further definition of it seems to be conceived as the analysis or articulation of the parts of the body. The Coans need not all have held exactly the same opinions. Some could have been more rigorous in making physiology depend on a simple nature philosophy and others less so, when they saw the body's complexity. Among the latter was perhaps Hippocrates. But the content of the Coan books, thus identified, does show Ionian nature philosophy pressing into the field of medical theory on a broad front.

The books in which Coan doctrine appear are: *Epidemics* I–III (really a single book), *Prognostic*, *Epidemics* II, IV and VI, *Humours*, *In the Surgery*, *Leverage*, *Fractures*, *Joints*, *The Nature of Bones*, *The Nature of Man* (attributed by Aristotle to Polybus, son-in-law of Hippocrates), *Airs, Waters, Places, The Sacred Disease, Epidemics* V and VII and also parts of *Aphorisms, Crises* and *Coan Prognoses,* which contain extracts or points borrowed from the longer works. This list is arranged in order of affinity to *Epidemics* I–III, the first-named book. Affinity covers manner, style and vocabulary, even in the surgical books which might seem of little relevance to the rest.

Cnidian books are much more strictly medical as we understand the term, and usually show little theoretical interest of a conscious kind. They are concerned with details and have very little structure, and never any literary quality. Their subjects in modern terms are regimen, pathology, gynaecology and embryology. Whereas Coan books err in being too speculative, Cnidian books from time to time have grotesque features such as curious readers have come to expect from the medicine of earlier ages; but others have a good claim to be scientific. Recognized as Cnidian by most authorities are the following books: *Regimen in Acute Diseases, Regimen in Health, Diseases* I, II, III and IV with *Seed, The Nature of Child, Affections, Internal Affections, The Nature of Woman, Diseases of Women, Sterile Women, Superfoetation, Excision of the Foetus, The Seven Months' Child* and *The Eight Months' Child, Diseases of Girls.*[79] Others may contain Cnidian material.

The other books are hard to assign to either of these schools or to any other, when so little is known in detail about the other schools. A distinct body of writings defined by its subject are those which concern medical ethics and etiquette, such as the *Oath, The Physician* and *Decorum*; they are generally judged to be among the later books.

CHAPTER IV

THE HIPPOCRATIC CORPUS

THE COLLECTION OF BOOKS which came to be named after Hippocrates has no more unity than any other medical library not devoted to some special subject. Nor do the individual books always confine themselves to one subject. For both these reasons it is justifiable in a history of Greek medicine to arrange most of the matter in the Corpus under headings which ignore the separation of one book from another and of one nameless author from another, though differences of view or approach can be noted. In spite of the differences between Hippocratic medicine and our own, therefore, the Hippocratic contribution to knowledge, theory and practice will be considered as far as possible under the categories of modern medicine.

MEDICINE DEFENDED AND DEFINED

Before we enter upon the departments of medicine, some books and passages in the Corpus referring to the whole art and science of healing deserve to be noticed. The medical profession in the fifth century was one of several which were forming themselves; it needed to be defined and defended against attack or annexation by nature philosophers and sophists in order both that it should continue and that it should enjoy professional respect.

The most important treatment of this theme is found in the book *Ancient Medicine* (*Περὶ ἀρχαιῆς ἰητρικῆς*), which begins by insisting, against the crude and vague speculations of the nature philosophers about the elements and the state of matter as they appear in the body, that medicine is an exciting and complex art in which some practitioners are good, some bad.[80]

This could not be the case if there were no art to learn.[81] Medicine arose because sick men cannot take the same food as healthy men, so that their dietetic needs had to be considered. Indeed the whole art of preparing human food could be included in it, since even healthy men need prepared food and cannot feed on raw things as animals do. Thus the art of cooking, which reduces the indigestible strengths of raw foods by means of heat, has saved many from illness and death throughout human history.[82]

Health consists of the proper blending in the body of humours of many kinds, which in their uncompounded state are strong and injurious. Medicine brings this about by suitable diet and regimen. To those who say that correct treatment can be given only by someone who knows, as Empedocles claimed to know, what man's constituents are and how he came into being, it should be answered that clear knowledge of nature can be derived from no source except medicine, which understands man in relation to what he eats and drinks.[83] (This claim is as exaggerated as the opposite one made by the nature philosophers. The two sides of the argument were continued in the seventeenth century and later by the physicians and the iatrophysicists and iatro-chemists in one phase of modern science.)

The other well-known defence of medicine written during this period is *The Art* (*Περὶ τέχνης*), which is written in the manner of a sophist, not of a physician, but makes some good points against the detractors of medicine.[84] These say, first, that cures are due to luck; secondly, that patients often recover without medical help; thirdly, that some patients die although they are treated by a physician; and fourthly, that physicians refuse to treat some illnesses.[85] The fundamental distinction asserted in *The Art* is between art and luck. It is allowed by both sides that some patients are cured, but because not all are cured the art is maligned and the cures are attributed to luck. Yet simply by becoming patients the sick acknowledge that there is more than luck in medicine and trust themselves to the art.[86] Another argument used in this defence is a sophism: that when those who have recovered without a physician have by chance correctly used a remedy that a physician would have recommended, they cannot claim to have been cured spontaneously, but only because of something definite, which is part of the art.[87] But it is obvious that, when an effective remedy or treatment is used which would have been prescribed, that fact alone does not constitute an achievement for the art, since the remedy was not knowingly and deliberately used by order of the physician.

Those who would deny the art because illnesses are sometimes fatal are putting no blame on the ill luck of the patient and all on the physician. They are in fact saying that while physicians may give wrong instructions, patients can never disobey orders. When a physician refuses to treat a hopeless case, he does so because the illness is too strong for the means at the disposal of medicine.[88] This ancient argument has regard only for the art and the practitioner, to save them from the discredit of false promises; it cannot anticipate the use of palliatives and pain-killing drugs, which rank as treatment though they cannot cure. *The Art* further praises medicine for its ability to use reason to deal with diseases that are not manifest to the eye, and to effect a cure if the disease has not gone too far to be overtaken. The evidence is in diagnostic signs such as peculiar urine or excrement.[89]

On another front superstition was the enemy, not so much attacking as needing to be attacked if the art of medicine was to be maintained. This appears in *The Sacred Disease* (*Περὶ ἱρῆς νούσου*) of which the first part consists of polemic against 'magicians, purifiers, charlatans and quacks' who claim superior knowledge of the disease, that is, epilepsy, but maintain an ancient tradition of superstition.[90] They use purifications and incantations, and forbid for ritual reasons the eating of many fish, animals and birds; these foods may indeed be bad for the sick, but the quacks prohibit them solely on the ground that epilepsy is of divine origin.[91] Anyone who can banish epilepsy by purification and magic can by similar means bring it on, as he can also bring down the moon, eclipse the sun and control the weather. These rites, if they are effective, show not the power of the gods but the power of man. If a particular god is to blame in epilepsy or in any of its manifestations, then by trying to purify the patient they are treating the divine influence as a defilement, and in fact showing impiety. For in fact it is godhead that purifies. The disease is no more divine and no more human than any other, in spite of its alarming appearance. It is brought about as an effect of weather and wind on certain constitutions, and both the weather and the human body are part of a divine order.[92] This attack on the diviners is like later rationalist attacks on superstition, but it is motivated by a form of natural theology which the author holds as part of his medical and scientific doctrine.

The same author appears to have written *Airs, Waters, Places* (*Περὶ ἀέρων ὑδάτων τόπων*), an essay in medical climatology in which he expresses his views on epilepsy in almost identical terms, though very briefly.[93]

ANATOMY

At this point, though the break is rather sudden, it seems best to begin applying the categories of modern medicine, always with due regard for the great differences in viewpoint between it and its ancient counterpart. The foundation of modern medicine is anatomy: the structures of the body are taught first in order that the processes of physiology and pathology may be located and surgery efficiently and safely carried out. Greek medicine on the other hand could not in this early period be based on anatomy, because human bodies were not dissected to reveal the interior organs or any other parts not easily visible. Dissection was forbidden on religious grounds, largely out of respect for the dead, and was not practised even on the corpses of foreign enemies or of criminals.[94] At most a body washed up on the seashore might be circumspectly examined, or aborted embryos and the bodies of exposed children might be cut open. Another reason was more practical: healing was practised on the sick and injured as occasion arose, and for such a purely clinical purpose anatomy seemed to be of little interest. None the less the Hippocratic books do contain anatomical passages which deserve attention. These will now be outlined with an occasional hint on their accompanying physiology before we reach physiology on its own account.

Places in Man (*Περὶ τόπων τῶν κατὰ ἄνθρωπον*), for instance, has a clearly anatomical title.[95] On the skeleton it has a few remarks, some of them odd. The skull is said to have in some cases three sutures, in others four; the three-sutured skull lacks one running backwards along the top.[96] On the brow ridge the bone is of double thickness. Vertebrae are more numerous in some people than in others, the greatest number being eighteen.[97] There are seven ribs joined at the spine and meeting again at the sternum. No floating ribs are mentioned. The clavicles are articulated to the sternum and the scapulae. The scapulae are articulated to the humeri on each side. Along each humerus two bony epiphyses run, one inside, the other outside, forming the articulation of the scapulae to the humeri. Lower down at the elbow the humerus is articulated in a natural cavity with the forearm at the olecranum. On the forearm four thin processes grow out from the bone, two above, two below, and are articulated at the elbow. The lower two are turned downward and both meet the upper process coming down from the humerus and form the joint. Lower down toward the hand the bone has an articulation; two of the long processes do not enter the joint, while the upper and lower join the bone of the hand. The hand has many articulations, as many as there are meetings of bones; the fingers also have their joints.[98]

At the hips there are two articulations called cups (κοτύλαι); the femora articulate there. The femora have two bony processes running along them which do not project anywhere. The femur bifurcates at its upper end, the inner piece having a rounded head which is received in the cup, the outer one and the ischium appearing low in the buttock. At the knee the femur likewise bifurcates, and the head of the tibia is engaged between its pieces as in a hinge-joint. Above this bone is the knee-cap (μύλη) which prevents the moisture of the flesh from entering the joint when it is extended. Along the tibia are two bony processes which end in the malleoli downward, but do not reach upwards to the knee-joint. The tibia articulates with the foot by the malleoli and again below them.[99] In the foot as in the hand, there are as many articulations as there are bones.[100] There are small articulations about the body which are not the same in all individuals, as there are small veins. Finally the mucus in joints is mentioned, which acts as a lubricant.[101] These descriptions of bones are on the whole accurate; the knowledge on which they rest would have come from some inspection of skeletons as well as from observation of living bodies, injured or uninjured. The writers of the surgical books would have had at least this much knowledge of the skeleton.

Another and a more prominent feature of Hippocratic anatomy consists in the accounts of vascular systems included in some of the books. From our point of view it is odd that so little notice is taken of the heart, though it is sometimes recognized as the centre of the vascular system, and the existence of pulsation was known. But, as will be shown when their physiology is treated, the Hippocratics had no conception of circulation, nor of the heart as a pump. Some of them regarded the brain as the most important part of the vascular system, for, though they came across individual nerves, they had no general idea of the nervous system. In fact they made use of the vascular system to explain the processes which we call neurological, for they could see that these required a system of channels ramifying about the body, and they knew of only one such system. In the Hippocratic accounts of blood-vessels the word φλέψ, usually translated 'vein', is used both for veins and for arteries, since these were not distinguished. Here it will be translated simply by 'vessel'.

In their general nature most of the Hippocratic plans of the vascular system are identical with the system of Diogenes already given.[102] The most primitive in character, whether or not it is the earliest in date, is that mentioned in *The Nature of Bones* (Περὶ ὀστέων φύσιος), and again by Aristotle in his *History of Animals*, where it is attributed to Syennesis, a pupil of Hippocrates.[103] In this there are two great vessels running from the eye along the eyebrow and through the lung under the breasts, one from the right eye to the left side of the body, and the other oppositely arranged. The vessel arising from the left eye runs through the liver to the right kidney and testicle. A vessel from the right breast runs to the left buttock, and *vice versa*. This curious crossing may originate from an observation which we should call neurological: that an injury on one side of the head affects nervous responses on the other side of the body. The system of Diogenes is certainly better than this.

The vascular system in *The Sacred Disease* closely resembles that of Diogenes, from which some scholars derive it, except that it revives Alcmaeon's view of the brain.[104] Vessels lead upward from all over the body to the brain; many of them are thin, but two are thick – clearly the *hepatitis* and *splenitis* of Diogenes. One section of the vein from the liver runs down on the right side of the body, close to the right kidney, through the loin and the inner part of the thigh and so down to the foot. This is called the hollow vein: its name is the original of our term *vena cava*. The other part of it reaches upward through the right diaphragm, putting out branches to the heart and the right arm, and then passes under the clavicle to the right side of the neck. It vanishes by the ear, sending off a thick branch to the brain and a thin one to the right ear and nostril. On the left side the *splenitis*, which is thinner, runs up and down in a similar manner, but passes through the spleen instead of the liver. Bilateral symmetry in this account is pressed further inside the trunk than nature allows. The lungs and their circulation seem to go unnoticed.

In *The Nature of Bones*, *The Nature of Man* (*Περὶ φύσιος ἀνθρώπου*) and Aristotle's *History of Animals*, and also in *Epidemics* (*'Επιδημίαι*), there are fragments of other notions of vascular systems. *The Nature of Bones* IX and *The Nature of Man* XI assert that there are four pairs of great vessels.[105] One pair runs from the back of the head, along the spine on either side to the buttocks and legs and so down to the feet. Bleeding for pains in the back and the buttocks must be carried out from this pair at the backs of the knees and the outside of the ankle. The second pair, called jugulars, come from the head near the ears and pass through the lumbar region to the testicles and thighs, and then by the inner edge of the knee at the back to the inner side of the ankles and feet. For lumbar pains and pains in the testicle bleeding must be performed behind the knee and at the ankle. The third pair runs from the temples by the neck to the scapulae, then to the lungs; thereafter the vessels cross before arriving at the spleen, the liver and the kidney, and finishing at the anus. The fourth pair runs from the front of the head and the eyes, under the clavicles to the upper and lower arms, wrists and fingers, and then returns by the palms and forearm to the elbow and armpit, thence to the spleen and the liver, and through the abdomen to the genitals. These vessels carry nourishment all over the body. Bleeding from them must be done according to the lie of them, and as far as possible from the site of the pain. Here we find therapeutic value assigned to an odd plan of the body's vessels.

The Nature of Bones X and *Epidemics* II have the two great vessels *hepatitis* and *splenitis* so arranged on either side that at one point a section of each runs inward to the heart to meet a section running outward to it.[106] Here at least it is recognized that the aorta and *vena cava* are not simply vessels that run up and down the body each in a single and uninterrupted course. More interesting is a puzzled reference to two stout cords (*τόνοι*) which run down from the brain under the great vertebra at the top and then traverse the neck on each side of the oesophagus and the *arteria* (*ἀρτηρίη*); after this they end at the meeting of the vertebra and the diaphragm, though they appear rather doubtfully to continue to the spleen and liver. Another pair of cords on either side originates from the vertebrae next to the clavicles, extends along the sides of the spine and reaches the ribs. They seem to pass through the diaphragm and the mesentery and there they apparently stop; but they are found again passing along the vertebrae until they come to an end at the extremity of the sacrum.

These cords are nerves, as they were later called. The Hippocratic author has no function for them, nor was he likely to find one, since the physiology of the period assigned nervous activity to the blood vessels. They are the cranial and sympathetic nerves of modern physiology, much easier to see than the familiar spinal nerves that run into the muscles.

Places in Man III has a system partly similar to the ones mentioned.[107] Several pairs of vessels originating in the head run about the head and downwards into the body in the familiar manner, but one pair converges to become the 'hollow vein' (*vena cava*) which runs between the trachea and the oesophagus, through the heart and diaphragm, before dividing in the lower body to enter the thighs and legs. The hollow vein also gives off symmetrical branches to left and right. Here we have one main vessel in the centre of the body which gives off branches, not two main vessels running parallel with relatively unimportant cross-junctions.

Finally, in *The Nature of Bones* XII–XIX we have the remarkable conception of the primal vessel (*ἀρχαίη φλέψ*), which runs downwards from the head and is always one in its main stem.[108] It has many lateral branches about the head, trunk and limbs, as would be expected, but combines some central organs and channels of the body in a bizarre manner, after which some of its branches return upwards, while others continue into the legs. In the thorax it has a very large branch which further subdivides to enter the heart by many openings. Thence it runs upwards in a tube (ἀρτηρίη) leading through the lungs to the mouth and containing little blood and much *pneuma*. In the lungs it has many ramifications and sometimes becomes cartilaginous, as also in the trachea. Downwards the primal vessel runs to the kidneys and testicles, while its main stem in men turns into the penis, and in women into the womb. Some paired branches run upwards again to the lungs, full of blood. But vessels coming out of the lungs carry thin and scanty blood, because the lungs have used it up, and these vessels are attached to the heart by the auricles as they enter it. The continuation of the gristly trachea by a blood vessel which eventually terminates in the penis suits some ancient physiological views, as we shall see. Our word trachea for windpipe is the Greek adjective τρηχείη, 'cartilaginous', referring to one section of this primal vessel, the ἀρτηρίη, which mingles blood and *pneuma*. Bronchi and blood vessels in the lungs are likewise confused. So far has physiological speculation replaced or supplemented observation unaided by dissection.

The short treatise *The Heart* (Περὶ καρδίης), on the other hand, shows close observation; indeed it is in a class by itself for accuracy.[109] It is thought to be later than most of the Corpus. The heart is described as pyramidal in form and dark red in colour. It is enclosed in a smooth envelope containing a little liquid from the lungs, so that it moves as if in a bladder. The liquid cools the heat of its vigorous beating. It is a very strong muscle because its flesh is densely packed. Under the one envelope are two separate ventricles (γαστέρες) which are quite different. The right ventricle lies prone, communicating with one vessel, and has more capacity than the other, though it leaves the end of the heart solid and is as if sewn on from the outside. The left ventricle is a little lower and in direct line with the left breast, and there the beating can be felt.

The wall of the heart is thick and is lodged in a fossa shaped like a mortar. It is softly enveloped by the lungs, which moderate its excess of heat since they are naturally cold, and further cooled by respiration. Both ventricles are rough inside, as if eaten away, the left more so than the right because of the greater amount of air and heat in it. The two ventricles appear to have no external orifices until the auricles are cut away at the top of the heart. Then the orifices of both are revealed. The thick vessel running upwards from one deceives the eye if it is cut. These the writer calls 'the sources of life for the nature of man'. The auricles are bellows which blow air into the heart, 'the work of a cunning artificer'. Vessels (φλεβία) provide respiration for the left ventricle and the *arteria* (ἀρτηρίη) for the right ventricle. Unseen valves (ὑμένες), some with a texture like spiders' webs, spread across the orifices of the ventricles and can close them tight; their form is semicircular. The left ventricle is fed by a fine extract from the blood. From the right ventricle a vessel conducts blood to the lungs to nourish them.

Much of this anatomy is very exact. The sigmoid valves with their outer edges attached to the inner walls of vessels and capable of meeting in the middle of the space, with no passage through their straight inner edges, are well observed. The pulmonary artery is indicated, though hardly the pulmonary vein. But does the account rest on any dissection of a human heart? If so, it must be that of an exposed infant and not an embryo, for during most of the prenatal period the heart has three chambers and not four.

Of the other organs the brain receives some anatomical description in *The Sacred Disease*, where it is said to be double like that of all animals, being parted down its centre by a thin membrane.[110] In *Head Wounds* (*Περὶ τῶν ἐν κεφαλῇ τρωμάτων*) the outer membrane, our *dura mater* just below the skull, is mentioned; it must never be wounded in trepanation.[111] *Places in Man* describes how two thin vessels run from the brain to the pupil through the enveloping membrane.[112] Of the two membranes, or *meninges*, the outer is thicker (the *dura mater*), while the inner (the *pia mater*) is thin and in contact with the brain; it is never the same again once it has been wounded. The brain is set more in the front of the head than in the back according to *Diseases* (*Περὶ νούσων*) II.[113] Though the liver is often mentioned, and also the spleen as enlarged in malaria, there is little description of either as a structure, and the same is true for other organs, except for the eye, described in *Fleshes* (*Περὶ σαρκῶν*), with its three envelopes, its pupil and its transparent fluid.[114] The anatomy of women will be treated under gynaecology. The anatomy of embryos, on the other hand, will be noticed under physiology, for in this case process is more important than structure.

PHYSIOLOGY

At a date when the internal organs were so little examined, their action in maintaining the processes of life could not often be followed directly. Speculation concerning the fluids and gases of the body proceeded vigorously, giving rise to the two bodies of doctrine most characteristic of Greek medicine and least resembling anything in our own, namely the theory of humours and the theory of *pneuma*. The mixture of humours in any man's body determined his permanent constitution and temperament as well as his health, and was affected both by diet and by weather or climate. The movement of *pneuma* about the body accounted for consciousness, whether in thought or in sensation and perception. The Coan school emphasized these doctrines more than did the others, but such thinking was found in all the schools. In our own medicine the nearest analogy to the humours is in the secretions of the ductless glands, but these are minute in quantity compared with the other liquids of the body, particularly with the blood which they enter. In *pneuma* we have an early forerunner of oxygen as it is now understood in its physiological action.

Though earlier writers, such as Alcmaeon, and also many writers in the Corpus assumed an indefinite number of humours, the important ones throughout the Corpus, and the only ones in *The Nature of Man*, are blood, phlegm and bile.[115] Bile is often said to be of two kinds, yellow and black. If we ask what observable fluids carried these names, the answer appears to be that phlegm is mucus in various passages but particularly in the nose. Yellow bile is what we still call bile, black bile is probably blood from internal haemorrhages which appears as a dark colouring in urine, vomit and excrement, and blood is what we call blood in its purest form. Much illness was ascribed to persistent dominance of one humour over the others, and in less extreme cases to permanent constitution and temperament. Black bile is more often mentioned than the others in morbid conditions, which would be natural if it was usually haemorrhage. But the humours are also regarded as permanent constituents of the body, so that no one of them was irredeemably morbid in itself. Particular organs are regarded as the sources of humours, though once released they pervade the body.

Ancient Medicine, as a dietetic book, has something to say of the humours, though not on any rigid classification. When we have a cold in the head there is a flux from the nostrils that is far more acrid than usual and may cause sores. Later, as the heat of the nostril ceases, the flux becomes thicker and less acrid with coction. And so it is wherever acrid and unmixed humours arise, as in the eyes during a cold. Similar discharges in the throat cause soreness, quinsy, erysipelas and pneumonia; they are at first salt, watery and acrid, and then become denser and riper as the fever declines.[116]

All complaints arise from 'powers' (*δυνάμιες*), that is, substances with active and causal properties: bitter yellow bile, causing nausea, burning and weakness, or pungent acidities, causing frenzy and gnawing of the bowel and chest. The suffering ends only with 'coction', when through mixture the properties change and a calm state follows. Some humours are subject to a self-induced change, as when sweet humours become acid.

The Sacred Disease in its positive exposition of the author's own doctrine gives a classic account of phlegm as a source of illness. Epileptics are said to inherit from their parents an excess of phlegm in the brain, which causes their disease – it does not attack the bilious. Even the embryo in such cases will have an excessive flux or deliquescence from the whole brain, and, as he grows after birth, a diseased head, because not enough of the liquid is ever purged in running sores or in superabundant saliva or mucus. The discharge of phlegm will cause, according to its direction, palpitation of the heart with difficulty in breathing because of the chill which it brings, diarrhoea in the bowels, and convulsions about the body if it enters the two great vessels and chills the blood or if it blocks the flow of vital *pneuma*. Fluxes are brought on by sudden changes of temperature, particularly when the brain is first heated and then chilled, either by sudden change of wind or weather or by walking into a hot room or out of it. The south wind in general favours the disease.[117] The brain may also be corrupted by bile so that the patient becomes maniacal, noisy and restless, and as his brain becomes heated may shout at night because of his dreams.[118]

There are typical examples of excess in the humours. In *Airs, Waters, Places*, almost certainly by the same author, the morbid effects of humoral excess appear again. In cities exposed to hot winds and sheltered from northerly ones the inhabitants have heads full of phlegm, and are poor eaters and drinkers with weak digestions; the women are unhealthy and subject to fluxes. In cities exposed to north winds the inhabitants are bilious rather than phlegmatic, sinewy, spare, with hard healthy heads, but costive and liable to internal lacerations. Cold waters make the women inclined to be barren with scanty menstruation. In cities exposed to east winds the people have better health, no doubt because the humours are in balance; in cities exposed to west winds, however, they have all manner of diseases because their weather is like autumn with great and unhealthy changes throughout the day, and, we should infer, unhealthy alternation of dominant humours. Marshy drinking water causes phlegmatic diseases, and water from snow and ice should, by contrast, produce bilious ones.[119]

These principles also constitute the theory of disease in *Epidemics*, in which the books have general sections on the weather at each season of the year, and also case-histories, most accurately observed, whose merits are quite independent of the authors' theory. The sections on prevailing weather are called καταστάσεις which is traditionally rendered 'constitutions'. The constitutions are those of the surrounding weather, not of the inhabitants of any place. The weather that favours one humour or another to the point of producing a morbid excess of it is described round the year.[120] The case-histories in the various books, on the other hand, make comparatively little explicit mention of the humours, partly no doubt because they concern immediately visible manifestations of illnesses and not speculations about their causes. Bile is much more often mentioned than phlegm, no doubt because the illnesses are mostly fevers in which the stomach and intestines are disordered. But there are also references to phlegm. The subject of humours is more explicitly treated in the book called *Humours* (*Περὶ χυμῶν*), which belongs closely with *Epidemics*, and also has connections with other books, particularly with *Airs, Water, Places.*[121] It is written in a very disjointed manner, like some books of *Epidemics*. The reader is told that he must know in what seasons humours break out, what diseases they cause in each season, and what symptoms they cause in each disease. He must know to what disease the physical constitution most inclines. For example a swollen spleen produces a certain effect, to which the constitution contributes something; so too with an evil complexion and with parching of the body. These considerations lead us into pathology, which will be treated later. Meanwhile the contributions of some other books to humoral theory must be noticed.

The Nature of Man states the classical doctrine of four humours, as accepted by Galen and perpetuated for many centuries after him. The constituents of man are blood, phlegm, yellow bile and black bile, each quite unlike the others in colour, in warmth or coldness, or in dryness or moisture. A different medicine will bring each one out of a man at any time or season: but, with continued dosing or purging directed at drawing out one, the others will eventually follow.[122] Phlegm, which is white, increases in winter; it is the coldest constituent in the body, as touch will show. This effect of winter can be seen from sputum, from nasal discharges, from white swellings and from the phlegmy diseases.[123] In spring phlegm remains strong in the body, but blood increases. As the cold relaxes and the rains come on, blood, which is moist and warm, increases through the showers and hot days, for it is akin to spring. This can also be seen from the dysentery and nasal haemorrhage that come in spring and summer, when men are hot and red.[124] In summer blood is still strong, but yellow bile rises in the body and increases until autumn.[125]

In autumn, which is hostile to its nature, blood diminishes but bile continues, and yellow bile is gradually replaced by black.[126] As winter comes on black bile is chilled and reduced, and gives way to phlegm.[127] Thus these elements, always present in the body, vary seasonally in amount because of heat, cold, dryness and moisture, and in each year one of the seasons is more powerful than the others. When one humour is excessive because of the season or from some other cause, treatment must be set against it. Most fevers come from bile. This is the most schematic of all the accounts of the humours.

Different from the morbid or seasonal dominance of one humour is its dominance in the permanent constitution as the temperament of a man. This distinction was not easy to press even in ancient times, but an important system of temperaments was set up, which was for centuries even more prominent than the doctrine of temporary dominance. To this we owe the familiar classification, phlegmatic, sanguine, choleric and melancholic, which is found in so much later literature in the Greek and Roman world and afterwards. But these terms as found in the Hippocratics are always directly linked to the doctrine of physical humours, and do not yet take on an almost separate life as psychological expressions. As constitutional types broadly defined, phlegmatic and bilious persons of both sexes, the former with soft, relaxed bodies and calm or sluggish dispositions, the latter dry and tense in body with excitable, energetic and often fierce natures, are assumed with variations throughout all books of the Corpus which have reason to distinguish physiques and constitutions. The humoral theory, in spite of its artificial appearance, underlies most of Hippocratic medicine. It has the same importance in the history of science as the doctrines of phlogiston or caloric in earlier stages of modern physics or chemistry.

The analogies are obvious between this ancient doctrine and modern observations on the action of the endocrine secretions which determine the slow or fast pace of living, the low or high excitability, the steadiness or the restlessness, and also the growth and the physical appearance of every human being.

The doctrine of *pneuma* or vital air developed in Hippocratic medicine under strong influence from the nature philosophers, particularly from Diogenes of Apollonia, already noticed for his physiological interests. Within the Corpus it was a favourite part of Coan medicine. It is well represented in *The Sacred Disease* and in *Airs, Waters, Places*. According to *The Sacred Disease* the great vessels running downward from the brain are also the vents of the body, drawing most of the air or *pneuma* to themselves, spreading it through the minor vessels about the body to cool it, and then breathing it out again. The breath cannot rest but moves up and down.[128] If it is caught anywhere, that part of the body where it is stopped becomes paralysed. This is shown when minor vessels are so compressed in lying or sitting that the breath cannot pass through them. For then a numbness seizes the man in that part.[129] Even here it is clear that air has its own life, which is expressed in continual movement. Self-movement, indeed, was almost the definition of life among Greek thinkers. Thus the life of the body is communicated to it by the air as a vital principle, not merely sustained by it as a necessary component, as in modern physiology. The observation of numbness is valid enough; we attribute this to the cutting off of the blood and all its ingredients.

On this view epilepsy is caused, as we noticed, by a general cutting off of the flow of air downwards from the brain through excess of phlegm. When a man takes in breath through the mouth or nostrils it first goes to the brain, after which most of it goes to the belly, though some reaches the lungs and some the vessels. The air which goes into the belly cools it but has no further use; the air that enters the cavity of the body and the brain, however, causes intelligence and movement of the limbs, so that when it is cut off the patient is speechless and senseless. Air stopped in the body rushes up and down, causing convulsions and pain; but when the vessels again admit it intelligence returns. Patients are attacked by epilepsy both when a north wind chills and condenses the air and when a south wind melts and diffuses it, for among the effects of these changes are fluxes of phlegm from the brain.

Air gives the brain its intelligence, so that the sense organs and the limbs act by its discernment; for it is the messenger to consciousness.[130] The inbreathed air, reaching the brain first, leaves its quintessence there: if it entered the body first, that, and not the brain, would have discernment, and the air would reach the brain hot and impure. This physiology accounts for the effects of the winds, varying in heat and humidity, which are asserted in *Airs, Waters, Places.* Modern physiology does allow the oxygen in the air to have these vivifying effects when it is carried about the body by the red corpuscles of the blood in chemical fixation, but it requires the nervous system to bring them about, using oxygen as a necessary means for its functioning. It agrees with *The Sacred Disease*, though on its own terms, in predicting the consequences when the brain is starved of oxygen.

The other full source for the theory of *pneuma* in this age is the rhetorical exercise *Breaths* (*Περὶ φυσῶν*).[131] This does indeed deal with air in the body, but as well as using the words *pneuma* and *aēr* (ἀήρ), it uses the word *phusa* (φῦσα), which we translated as 'gas' when considering the influence of Egyptian theory. This variety of terms indicates a confusion which is surely deliberate. The aim is to use these words for air or gas as if they had the same meaning, and so to argue that all diseases have one origin, which is also a necessity of life.

Diseases, it is claimed, have all the same fashion, essence or cause, though the seat varies. Along with food and drink, air (πνεῦμα) is the third thing that nourishes the body. πνεῦμα in the body is called φῦσα, but outside it ἀήρ. ἀήρ, air, is the most powerful thing in nature. It is present everywhere, but invisible, nourishing the fire of the sun and maintaining the life of aquatic creatures, which inhale it as something present in water.[132] Breathing is continuous for all mortal creatures. Since they all participate in air, it is likely that maladies arise from this source. Indeed all diseases arise from air.

The commonest disease is fever, which is associated with other diseases. Fevers are either epidemic, common to all, or they are due to bad regimen in individuals. Air can be infected with pollutions hostile to the human race as a whole. In individuals fever can arise from an excessive amount of food without exercise, and from excessive variety of it. All food is accompanied into the body by wind (πνεῦμα) in greater or less quantity. This can show itself immediately in belching, but over a longer period the lower belly can become obstructed, and breaths (φῦσαι) can spread through all the body, chilling the parts that are most full of blood and causing a shiver to pass through the whole body owing to this chilling.[133]

As the blood tries to escape the chills and shivers it rushes to the viscera, causing the sick man to shake with the unequal amounts of blood in different parts. Diseases of the intestines such as ileus and tormina are equally due to the pressure or piercing action of wind (πνεῦμα), and fomentations are used to relieve these pains.[134] Haemorrhages of the chest arise when the vessels of the head are too full of air and compress the blood. The thinnest part of the blood then escapes downwards into the chest. Thus blood, and also phlegm, cause all manner of local pains in the chest and throat.[135] Fluxes of phlegm, water or melted flesh cause dropsy.[136] Copious breaths rushing through the whole body cause apoplexy.[137] Breaths also cause epilepsy, and blood disturbed by them impairs intelligence.[138] In this outline of a very odd book, those who suffer from flatulence will recognize here and there their own subjective feelings. Feelings, indeed, must have contributed largely to diagnosis and pathology as the Hippocratics saw them.

The normal physiology of organs is very little treated in any explicit fashion in the Corpus, though the writers necessarily knew something of the function of the stomach, intestines, kidney and bladder. The action of the liver and gall-bladder in storing bile is correctly diagnosed in *Diseases*.[139] In the same book the water of the body is less correctly said to have its seat in the spleen, and blood to be manufactured in the heart and transmitted elsewhere through the vessels, but apparently in a gentle flow. As we have seen, the action of the heart as a pump was not understood, though the pulse was noted, and the circulation was still less known. In *The Heart* the lungs are regarded as a cooling apparatus for the hot heart. [140] Even the brain, though Alcmaeon and his followers in the Corpus so well understood its importance, is treated as a sort of gland in *Glands* (*Περὶ ἀδένων*), where its function is to dispatch moisture about the body.[141] In *Fleshes* it is quaintly called 'the metropolis of the cold and glutinous', enclosed in a tunic of membranes and containing fatty parts.[142] Though the positive functions of some organs were only understood dimly or not at all, there are constant references to pains and discomforts felt in them. From such morbid states as are described it would be hard indeed to infer the healthy action of these organs.

None the less, *Fleshes* is the nearest approach in the Corpus to a general physiology. It begins with a paragraph on heat, which is called immortal, the universal intelligence, seeing, knowing and understanding all things both present and future. Heat in this account recalls the ever-living fire of Heraclitus, and the same claims are made for it that we have seen made for air in other books. In the cosmogonic process, one element, the purest fire, reached the outermost circumference of the world to become aether. Far below it a cold and dry but mobile element settled, that which we call earth, though it has some fire in it. A third element, rather warm and humid, settled below the aether. A fourth, not named, settled near the earth. It was humid and relatively dense; clearly this is water.[143]

From these elements, described entirely in the manner of nature philosophy and considered as inherently hot or cold, the author tries to constitute the human body. Some of the hotter patches of earth turned to bone when they lacked moisture; others, retaining some moisture, were not so far hardened and became sinew. Others again which were glutinous and had more cold in them became membranes; others, chillier still, became liquids. The hollow vessels of the body, throat, gullet, stomach and intestines, became so because their glutinous part was continually roasted and hardened. This account is an attempt to trace the origin behind the continuing effect of heat of the various tissues of the body from the materials found in the outer world. It can be called a larval beginning of biochemistry, made without any knowledge of cells and their activities, which only the microscope would reveal, or any conception of the chemical evolution by which these complex tissues would arise.[144]

Though the description of the brain in *Fleshes* is far from adequate, there are some interesting points. The brain not only forms a membrane about it, but further forms the bony skull as the heat continues. It is indeed claimed in modern physiology that the nerve cells have a chemical effect on surrounding tissues which leads to the formation of bone in some cases. The author emphasizes that the spinal marrow comes down from the brain and is of the same material, having much less fatty and glutinous material in it than the marrow of the bones, which is properly so called, and having also membranes about it as the brain has.

The heart, containing much glutinous and cold material, is turned by heat into a hard and tenacious kind of flesh. The greatest heat in the heart is where the hollow vein is attached – an odd statement because it is the other vessel, the *ἀρτηρίη*, which carries air about the body. Air is thus supplied to the body in its parts and organs. The heart and its vessels move continually: because it is the hottest organ the heart draws air into itself. Some connection is evidently felt by the author between the heart and respiration, for he mentions the *ἀρτηρίη*, the imaginary vessel which begins as the windpipe and continues as part of the vascular system through the heart. This vessel combines the roles played in modern anatomy by the windpipe and bronchi, the pulmonary vein, and the aorta, which distributes oxygenated blood through the arteries. The continual movement of the heart and its vessels is clearly the heartbeat and the pulse. But there is still no approach to any conception of regular circulation, including the return of blood to the heart.

In its movement the heart continually attracts air to maintain its heat as the flame of a lamp does, whether or not the draught is perceptible. The lungs are formed next to the heart, which heats moist and glutinous matter and gradually dries it up in a foamy state, so that they become spongy and full of small vessels. The cold element in this glutinous mass is melted into liquid, and the most glutinous part dried into a membrane. The liver arises from moisture heated without glutinous and fatty components. The spleen is formed with cold and glutinous elements, the latter composing its fibres. The kidneys are composed of a little glutinous material and a little heat, with much cold, which causes coagulation. Thus cold fixes and coagulates materials and makes flesh of them, while the glutinous element forms hollow vessels for containing blood or other moisture. Similar explanations are given for the formation of joints, nails, teeth and hair. The process of formation was no doubt conceived to begin in the embryo for all generations except the first, which was thought to have originated from the earth by other means.[145] Before the development of chemistry in modern times, there could be no fundamental improvement in these notions, but it is easy to see what problems were before the author's mind. They were those of the origin and differentiation of living matter.

FEMALE PHYSIOLOGY, REPRODUCTION AND EMBRYOLOGY

Little is said in the Hippocratic Corpus on the distinctive anatomy and physiology of the female body. From the scientific point of view this is surprising, but given the practical origin and concerns of medicine it is natural enough, for the subject arises mainly in a clinical context, whether in the treatment of women's illnesses or in obstetrics. So in our own time the term gynaecology is not used except in a clinical sense; and, as we shall see, on gynaecology in its modern sense the Hippocratic material is very full. On the related subject of reproduction the Hippocratic views appear strange indeed to the modern mind, which has had the benefit of the microscope. The same strangeness will appear in the Hippocratic views on heredity, where our own knowledge depends on more than the microscope alone. But on the later growth of the embryo, which would sometimes have been illustrated by premature birth, the Corpus presents views that seem to us much less odd.

There is no set account in any Hippocratic book of the anatomy of the female organs of generation – or at least of those too far within the body to be seen or reached without the dissection of cadavers, which was forbidden, or operation, which was beyond the surgery of the time. There is no mention, for instance, of a Caesarian section in the Corpus. Clinical experience in attempting to cure or mitigate diseased conditions of the vagina or the womb necessarily provided some knowledge of their anatomy, but the Hippocratics, in their circumstances, remained ignorant of the ovaries and Fallopian tubes and therefore of the causes and mechanism of menstruation.

At the beginning of *The Nature of Woman* (*Περὶ γυναικείης φύσιος*), really a clinical book, there is a classification of women's constitutions. Some women are said to be white, humid and subject to fluxes and others dark, dry and dense of flesh, while an intermediate class is ruddy.[146] In *Airs, Waters, Places* similar differences are attributed to phlegmatic and bilious constitutions in women, and to the northern or southern exposures of the localities where they live.[147] In clinical practice various distortions of the womb from its proper position are mentioned, as in *The Nature of Woman* and *Diseases of Women* (*Γυναικεῖα*); the physicians treating them would need to know what that position was.[148] The same physicians treated prolapse, for which that knowledge was equally necessary.

But strange beliefs persisted, as that the right side of the womb was warmer than the left and so produced male embryos, which matured more quickly than female. These were inherited from the nature philosophers, and are found, for instance, in *Epidemics* II and in *Prorrhetic* (*Προρρητικά*) II.[149] It has even been suggested that the womb was once thought to have two compartments, as in some animals. Between two distinct cavities such a difference in temperature and conditions would have seemed more conceivable. Lactation is explained in *The Nature of Child* (*Περὶ φύσιος παιδίου*) by the pressure of the enlarged womb in late pregnancy on the other tissues, which concentrates fatty material in the breasts and makes them swell.[150] But such an accumulation of oddments does not even outline an anatomy and physiology of the female body.

More instructive is the theory of reproduction and heredity that is stated or assumed with little variation in the Coan books *Airs, Waters, Places* and *The Sacred Disease* and in the Cnidian *Generation* (*Περὶ γονῆς*) and *The Nature of Child.* In *Airs, Waters, Places* a doctrine of semen and heredity is brought in to explain the character of the Macrocephals or Long-heads. Their heads were once forced into a long shape by binding in infancy, but by the author's time their heads had become long by heredity, so that binding was no longer necessary to produce this shape, which was considered a mark of nobility. Repeated binding through the generations had made this shape a part of their nature. This happened because seed comes from all parts of the body, healthy seed from the healthy parts, diseased seed from diseased parts. If baldness, grey eyes, squinting and other physical features are inherited, what prevents a long-headed parent from having a long-headed child?[151] In *The Sacred Disease* the same argument of seed collected from all parts of the parental body is used to prove that epilepsy can be hereditary.[152]

In *Generation* it is said that semen comes from all the liquid in a man's body, being the most active part of it. That is why ejaculation leaves us weak. Vessels and sinews (*νεῦρα* – this can hardly yet mean nerves) reach from all parts of the body to the genitals. The liquid becomes foamy by agitation, and its most active and fatty element enters the spinal marrow. The brain also discharges liquid into the spinal marrow; this view is the same as Alcmaeon's, that semen is a drop from the brain. The liquid passes through the kidneys to the testicles and so by a special channel, not the urinary one, to the penis. The flow is stopped in eunuchs because the channel is destroyed by castration. Those who have had incisions made in the vessels behind the ears have a main contribution cut off from the sum of the semen, so that they are infertile.[153] The same operation with the same result is also mentioned among the Scythians in *Airs, Waters, Places*.[154] In male infants the seminary vessels are small and blocked; in female infants the same cause prevents menstruation. This implies that menstruation is regarded as a flow of female seed.

Both sexes have both male and female seed.[155] The sex of the infant is determined by the greater strength of male, or of female, seed that goes to the engendering at the time. The likeness of a child to its parents is explained by the same mingling of seed from all parts of both parents' bodies. Mutilation in the parent is likely to cause a corresponding defect in the child, but a womb that is not large enough may cause further malformation.[156]

The mingled seed remains in the womb and is steadily warmed and draws breath into itself. The mother's breathing also draws in breath which is cooler than the breath that the seed or embryo already has. The parcel of seed develops a crust like baking bread as the breath enters it, retaining a hole through which to take in further breath. This is evidently the umbilical cord. The embryo so formed grows by nourishment from the mother's blood, and while the blood is used for this purpose there is no menstruation.

Other membranes grow round the first crust or envelope to be formed.

Nourished with this blood the flesh grows, with the umbilical cord always distinct from it in order to keep up respiration and growth.[157] When the membranes are fully developed they constitute the chorion. The growing flesh separates itself into the parts of the body, like joining to like, dense to dense, rare to rare, wet to wet. The bones are coagulated and hardened by heat. The whole body articulates itself like a tree, but mostly the outermost and the innermost parts: head, arms, legs, sinews, nose, ears, eyes, genitals, viscera. Respiration begins by the mouth and nose, the belly fills itself with air and the intestines shut off the air entering by the cord. Passages are opened to the anus and from the bladder outward. Finally the hair and nails grow. It is respiration that maintains this articulation, while all the material is supplied by the mother's body. An elaborate comparison is made with the growth of plants. Another comparison, more illuminating, is made with the growth of a chick within the egg, of which the stages can be observed by breaking open on successive days during incubation each one of twenty eggs all laid on the same day. On the analogy of the chick, it is argued that the human foetus brings on its own birth by agitating and breaking the membranes when its food is exhausted.[158] The birth of twins is explained by a variety of folds or recesses in the womb, which receive separate parcels of seed and develop them into distinct individuals, each with its own membranes and placenta. In a pair of twins one can be male and the other female because of a difference in the relative strength of the combined seeds.[159]

Decided views on premature birth are found in the linked books *The Seven Months' Child* (*Περὶ ἑπταμήνου*) and *The Eight Months' Child* (*Περὶ ὀκταμήνου*).[160] At the end of the sixth month of gestation the child is thought capable of surviving birth, though only a few do so. But children have a better chance of surviving if they are born during the seventh month than during the eighth. During the eighth month the foetus moves down into another position, dragging the placenta with it and causing discomfort to the mother, as women will confirm. A child born during this time will be blind and lame and will not live. If a child is born at the beginning of the ninth month it will be hard to rear, after being ill in the womb. The most healthy time for birth is at the end of the ninth month. The book called *Superfoetation* (*Περὶ ἐπικυήσιος*) is from its first paragraph a mixed compendium of obstetrical lore and hints on conception.[161]

The account of reproduction and heredity that emerges from these books is sensible enough, given the authors' necessary ignorance of some essential facts. The theory of pangenesis, as it is called, was a natural one to hold before the exclusive concentration of reproductive cells in the testicles and ovaries was shown.[162] This separation isolates the sperms and the ova from all effects of the environment felt by the rest of the body. It was natural for the Hippocratics to hold, in consequence, a strong form of Lamarck's opinion that characters acquired by the parent in his lifetime would be transmitted to the child. They could not make our distinction between the phenotype and the genotype.

The importance of the placenta in maintaining the life and growth of the foetus is well appreciated, and so is the shock of a changed environment which the child receives at birth.

CLINICAL DESCRIPTION AND PATHOLOGY

After so much consideration of biological theory and medical science, we come to the strictly clinical aspect of medicine. In any attempt to understand illness there are two elements which vary in relative importance according to the stage that medicine has reached. One is to observe the beginning and progress of the illness in all necessary detail, as shown by the patient's external appearance, by his behaviour, and by such manifestations as unusual breathing, sweating, excretion and temperature. The other is to try to discover the causes for this sequence of morbid symptoms, to establish what is in fact happening inside his body. Hippocratic medicine excelled in clinical observation, including close attention to such things as excrement and urine, so that even in our time medical men are moved to admiration. Like all other medicine until the last two or three centuries, the Hippocratic science was continually hindered in its attempt at causal explanation and pathology by the lack of such things as thermometers, microscopes and chemical tests of blood, urine and saliva, not to speak of more sophisticated aids.

The use of such scientific equipment is with us an important part of diagnosis, particularly of differential diagnosis, which it can confirm. Diagnosis in ancient times had to proceed by the accumulation and classification of external signs. In spite of much intellectual subtlety, this was not always very useful, and the Coan school, as we saw, preferred to give a prognosis of the likely course of an illness based on previous experience and not distracted by too many refinements. Thus *Prognostic* (*Προγνωστικόν*) and other books, which we shall now examine, are close studies of the visible process of disease undertaken for future guidance. Mostly they are not therapeutic; even in case-histories they do not usually say what treatment was applied. They are concerned particularly with diseases involving fever.

At the beginning of *Prognostic* the physician is advised to examine the face of his patient to see whether it is like the faces of healthy people and like its usual self. Unlikeness to these will be the most dangerous sign, as in the following points: nose sharp, eyes hollow, temples sunken, ears cold and contracted with their lobes turned outward, the skin about the face hard, tense and parched, and the colour of the whole yellow or black. He must go on to enquire whether the patient has been sleepless, whether his bowels have been very loose, and whether he suffers from hunger. The danger will be less if any of these things is confessed. If the face has this appearance the crisis comes after a day and a night. But if none of these things is confessed and there is no recovery within this period it is a sign of death. If the disease has lasted more than three days with the face having these characteristics the same enquiries must be made. The eyes must particularly be noticed. If they shun the light, weep without reason, or are distorted or unequal in size, if the whites are red or livid or show black vessels, if there is rheum round the eyeballs, if they are restless or protruding or very sunken, or if the whole complexion of the face is changed, these are bad or even fatal symptoms. If in sleep the whites appear when the lids are closed, and there has been no diarrhoea or purging and no habit of sleeping with eyes half-closed, this is an unfavourable, indeed very deadly, symptom. If in addition the eyelid, lip or nose is bent, death is close at hand. It is also a deadly sign if the lips are loose, hanging, cold or very white.

There is not of course space to quote the rest with the same particularity as this sample, but there are other points worth mentioning. There are sleeping postures which portend no good: lying on the back with arms and legs stretched out, bending forward and slipping towards the foot of the bed, lying with the mouth open or on the back with folded legs.[163] Wishing to sit when the disease is at its height is bad, especially in pneumonia.[164] Grinding of the teeth in fevers signifies madness and death.[165] In acute fevers it is a deadly sign to move the hands before the face, to hunt in the empty air, to pluck nap from the bedclothes, pick up bits or snatch chaff from the walls.[166] Rapid respiration indicates pain or inflammation above the diaphragm, slow respiration delirium.[167]

Sweating is good on critical days and when it occurs all over the body. Sweats round the head and neck only, however, indicate death in acute fever and in a milder fever long illness.[168] Dropsies resulting from acute diseases are all unfavourable.[169] Stools are best when soft and consistent and passed at the usual time.[170] Urine is best when the sediment is white, smooth and even throughout. If it is sometimes clear but sometimes contains a white deposit the illness will be longer and more dangerous. Reddish urine with smooth reddish sediment is good. Mealy or flaky sediments are bad. Thin white sediments are all bad. Clouds suspended in the urine are good when white, but bad when dark. Thin and yellowish-red urine is a sign that the disease is unripened, that the humours are still acid or bitter and not yet in a stable and healthy mixture. The more fatal kinds of urine are fetid, dark and thick in adults, but watery in children. Sometimes urine contains clouds because the bladder is diseased, and in this case the symptom does not indicate general unhealthiness. Sputum is bad if it is yellow, white, viscous and globular, pale green, frothy or dark.[171] It is always bad if it does not relieve the pain.[172] Empyema of the lungs is treated at length.[173] Apart from the sputum, continuous fever and copious sweats are mentioned; the eyes become sunken, the cheeks flushed, the fingers hot and the feet swollen, while the body is blistered in many places, and the appetite fails. Pain and dyspnoea at the beginning are signs of an early breaking; milder pain and other signs of proportionate mildness indicate a later breaking.[174] Pains with fever in the lower body are mortal if they then attack the diaphragm.[175] Hardness and pain in the bladder with continuous fever are very serious; but the disease is relieved by the passing of purulent urine with a white sediment.[176] The notions of critical days and *apostasis* are introduced here, but they will be discussed later under pathology.

There is little attempt at a clinical picture; the author even says that many diseases which have names are not mentioned by them in the *Prognostic*. The symptoms that are mentioned are given as indications of crisis, not as defining the disease.

The books of *Epidemics* are full of examinations of this kind, and from time to time have general pronouncements like those of *Prognostic*. In *Epidemics* I the author declares that he has framed his judgments from the common nature of all men and the peculiar nature of each patient, from the regimen and from the physician who prescribed it, and also from the constitution of the weather in each region. He has observed the customs, mode of life, practices and ages of patients; also their talk, manner, silence, thoughts, sleep, sleeplessness, the nature and time of dreams, pluckings, scratchings, tears, exacerbations of the illness, stools, urine, sputa, vomit; the antecedents and consequents of each successive disease; *apostasis* to a fatal issue or to a crisis; rigor, chill, coughs, sneezes, hiccoughs, breathing, belching, flatulence, silent or noisy, haemorrhages and haemorrhoids.[177] The continuous observation of the patient implied in any attempt to follow this method would of course have been impossible for one physician. For this, as for regular application of remedies throughout the twenty-four hours, some form of nursing would be required. What this may have been will be discussed later under therapy.

The title *Epidemics* as we use the word suits some of the fevers well enough, and also the background of 'constitutions' or set conditions of weather. But in the later books of the group, which are not worked up fully into the form shown by the earlier ones, there is much more miscellaneous and individual material, some of it hard to connect with general conditions or with humoral theory. There is therefore much to be said for one interpretation of the word *epidēmiai* (ἐπιδημίαι) – not visitations of widespread disease in an area, but the writers' visits to the region.[178] Regions such as Thasos are mentioned as the scene of these physicians' travels, which on this view would have been undertaken to gain wider experience than they would have gained at home.[179]

The accumulation of detail in the seven books of the *Epidemics* is so great that only a few of the most notable case-histories can be quoted. These can be supplemented with some other jottings of great interest, which would certainly not be relevant to case-histories of acute fever in an epidemic. Fever, as was usual for centuries to come, is treated as a disease in itself, not as a reaction of the body.

> Philiscus lived by the wall. He took to his bed; on the first day, acute fever; he sweated; night uncomfortable. On the second day, general exacerbation, and later had a good movement of the bowels by a small clyster; night restful. On the third day, early and until midday he seemed to be rid of the fever, but toward the evening, acute fever with sweating; thirsty, dry tongue, black urine; night uncomfortable, did not sleep, completely out of his mind. On the fourth day, general exacerbation; dark urine; night more comfortable with urine of better colour. On the fifth day about midday a slight bleeding of unmixed blood from the nose; urine varied, with round bodies suspended in it, resembling semen, and scattered about; they did not settle. When a suppository was applied, scanty excreta were passed with flatulence. Night painful, short snatches of sleep, talking, raving; extremities everywhere cold and would not warm up again; dark urine, a little sleep toward dawn; speechless; cold sweat; extremities livid. On the sixth day about midday he died. His breathing throughout was as if he were recollecting to do it, rare and large. His spleen was raised in a round swelling; cold sweats throughout. Exacerbation on even days.[180]

This was surely a very bad case of malaria, a disease which appears to have struck Greece as an epidemic for the first time late in the fifth century.

> Meton was seized with fever and painful heaviness in the loins. On the second day, after a rather copious draught of water, he had a good motion of the bowels. On the third day heaviness of the head; stools thin, bilious and rather red. On the fourth day, general exacerbation; slight bleeding twice from the right nostril; night uncomfortable; stools as on the third day; urine rather dark; darkish clouds floating in it, spread out, not settling. On the fifth day, violent bleeding from the left nostril; sweat; crisis. After crisis, sleeplessness; his speech wandered; urine thin and rather dark. He had his head bathed, slept, recovered his reason. He suffered no relapse, but had several haemorrhages from the nose after the crisis.[181]

This fever was at least not malaria, for it did not return, nor was the spleen enlarged.

> Walking about, Crito in Thasos felt a violent pain in the great toe. He took to his bed on the same day with shivering and nausea; recovered a little warmth, was delirious at night. On the second day he had a swelling of the whole foot, which was rather red about the ankle, with distention and black blisters; acute fever, mad delirium. Motions from the bowels, unmixed, bilious and rather frequent. He died on the second day from the beginning.[182]

Was this a very severe case of blood-poisoning? But no cut or bite is mentioned.

> The wife of Dromeades, after giving birth to a daughter when everything else had gone normally, on the second day was seized with rigor; acute fever. On the first day she had begun to feel pain in the hypochondrium; nausea, shivering, restlessness; did not sleep during the succeeding days. Respiration rare, large, and breath drawn in again suddenly. On the second day after her rigor, she had a good action of the bowels. Urine thick, white, turbid, like urine which has settled, stood a long time, and then been stirred up. It did not settle. At night she

did not sleep. On the third day rigor about midday; acute fever, urine similar; pain in the hypochondrium, nausea; night uncomfortable; she did not sleep. She had a cold sweat all over the body, but quickly recovered warmth. On the fourth day she felt a slight relief of the pain about the hypochondrium, but heaviness about the head with pain; was rather comatose, bled a little from the nostrils. Tongue dry; thirsty; scanty urine, thin and oily; slept a little. On the fifth day, thirsty; nausea; urine similar, no movement of the bowels; but about midday she had much delirium and then quickly recovered her reason. She rose but became rather comatose; slight chilling, slept at night; was delirious. On the sixth day, early, she had a rigor, but quickly recovered warmth, and sweated all over; extremities cold, was delirious. Respiration large and rare. Soon convulsions began from the head. She died soon after.[183]

From its sudden onset after the childbirth, this should be puerperal fever.

Outside the case-histories, *Epidemics* II has a vivid picture of patients suffering from ardent fevers and phrenitis. These came on early in the spring after the cold spells, and the sufferers displayed acute and fatal symptoms.[184] The ardent fevers had the following constitution. At the beginning coma, nausea, shivering, acute fever, no excessive thirst nor delirium; slight bleeding at the nose. The exacerbations in most cases came on even days, and about that time there was loss of memory with prostration and speechlessness. The feet and hands of these patients were always colder than normal, but particularly so at the time of the exacerbation. Slowly and unhealthily they recovered their warmth, came to their senses again and conversed. Either the coma held them, continuous and without sleep, or they were wakeful and in pain. Most of them had disordered bowels, and crude, thin, copious stools. Urine was copious and thin and had no critical or favourable sign. Nor did any other critical sign appear, such as haemorrhages or abscession. They died, not in a uniform fashion, at the crisis; many of them were speechless and many sweating.

The cases of phrenitis were similar, without thirst or mad delirium; the patients died heavy in the head with a dull stupor. The ardent fever which had periodical exacerbations may have been a virulent malaria. Phrenitis is on no modern list of diseases; its name must once have indicated an affliction of the diaphragm, which among the early Greeks was regarded as the seat of thought. Later, perhaps, when the brain was so regarded, it may have meant a fever of the brain.

The same book again, in its second 'constitution', has a classic description of pulmonary tuberculosis, a disease which is very prominent in the Corpus.[185] It is called the most serious and difficult of all the diseases of the year. In the winter many people suffered from it, of whom some took to their beds and others died without doing so. In spring most of those in bed died of it, but among those who remained alive the persistent cough diminished during the summer. In the autumn all of these took to their beds again and many died. Most of them endured long illnesses.

Sudden aggravation of the disease showed itself in this way: frequent shivering; in many cases continuous acute fever; sweats that were unseasonable, copious and cold during the whole illness; considerable chilling, succeeded by very imperfect recovery of warmth; bowels constipated in various ways and then quickly loosening, and always violently loose toward the end, as all the humours from the lungs made their way downwards; abundant urine of a bad kind, and malignant wasting. The coughs throughout were frequent and brought up quantities of concocted and liquid sputum, but without too much pain. There was little sore throat or distress from salt humours. The fluxes from the head were viscid, white, moist and frothy. But the worst symptom was the distaste for food or drink with nourishment; the victims had no thirst. They were heavy in the body and comatose. Most had swellings which turned to dropsy. They had fits of shivering and delirium near death.

The physical character of the tuberculous was: skin smooth, rather white, lentil-coloured or reddish; a bright-eyed, leucophlegmatic look, shoulder blades projecting like wings. The women were the same. Where the complexion was atrabilious or sanguine they were attacked by ardent fevers, phrenitis and dysenteric troubles. The young and phlegmatic ones had tenesmus; the bilious had chronic diarrhoea with acid, greasy stools.

A few other examples, given in summary, will illustrate the miscellaneous variety of illnesses or injuries recorded in *Epidemics*.

In Thasos some patients had swellings beside one or both ears, which subsided without causing harm or suppurating. They were flabby, big, spreading and without inflammation or pain. The sufferers were usually young men who frequented the wrestling school or the gymnasium. Sooner or later painful inflammation occurred in one testicle or in both, with fever or without it.[186] This has been recognized as the first known mention of mumps.

A shoemaker, making holes in a sole, pricked himself above the knee, and sank in the instrument about a finger's length. No blood flowed and the wound soon closed, but the whole thigh swelled up and so did the groin and the flank. He died on the third day.[187] This would have been blood-poisoning.

A man who was wounded in the groin by an arrow was unexpectedly saved. The point was too deeply lodged to be extracted, but there was no haemorrhage or inflammation, nor was the patient lamed. The point was still embedded when the writer saw the man six years later; it must have been lodged between tendons without cutting vein or artery.[188] This is one of the few Hippocratic passages where a difference between veins and arteries is recognized.

A man who was struck from behind by a sharp dart a little below the neck had a wound which did not look serious because it did not go deep. But some time later when the point had been extracted the patient was seized with backward-bending convulsion like those of opisthotonus. His jaws were locked, and any liquid that he attempted to swallow was returned through his nostrils. He died on the second day.[189] A clear case of tetanus; did the infection come from the original wound or from the surgeon's work?

A man fell wounded in the head by a Macedonian's sling stone. By the third day he had lost his power of speech and was tossing with a mild fever. There was a slight pulsing at the temples. He could hear nothing. He lost his reason, and was very restless. On the fourth day moisture came out round his forehead, under his nose, and as far as his chin. He died.[190] Was this damage to the brain? But the point of wounding is not clear, nor is there any mention of injury to the skull.

In a man who was wounded with a javelin in the liver the whole surface of the skin took on the colour of a corpse; his eyes were sunken, he tossed on his bed. He was wounded at dawn and died at dusk.[191]

These cases show that the Coan physicians took the opportunities for gaining experience afforded by warfare. The next case is provided from an accident at sea.

The superintendent of freight from a big boat had the index finger and the lower bone of his right hand crushed by the anchor. Inflammation, gangrene and fever followed. He swallowed a moderate purge; he felt a moderate degree of heat and pain; part of his finger fell away. After seven days there was a satisfactory discharge. Then he complained of his tongue; he could not articulate anything properly. The prognosis was that an opisthotonus would come. His jaws came together with a hard thrust; next his neck was affected. On the third day his whole body was bent backward, with sweating. The sixth day after the prognosis he died.[192] This is one of the clearest cases of tetanus coming on after the patient had survived other dangers.

Another case from warfare is the following. Tychon at the siege of Daton was wounded in the chest by a catapult bolt. Soon after he was seized with a noisy fit of laughing. The physician who extracted the shaft seems to have left some piece of wood in the diaphragm. The physician administered a clyster and a purgative in the evening. After a painful night the patient next day appeared better to his physician and others. The prognosis was that when a convulsion came he would die promptly. The next night his condition was painful, he could not sleep. He lay most of the time on his belly. On the third day in the morning he was seized with convulsions and died.[193] An interesting point is that the diaphragm was convulsed separately in the laughing fit. Otherwise it is like the other cases of tetanus.

Some cases were noted for their mental symptoms. A certain

Nicanor was eager to drink at parties but was frightened of the flute girl when she began playing. He was beset by terrors, and said that he could hardly contain himself at night. But if he heard the sound by day he was not disturbed at all. This remained with him a long time.[194] Democles, who was with him, seemed to have his sight obscured and to be unable to tense his body; he would never pass near a precipice or over a bridge, but he could walk along the ditch itself.[195] This continued to happen for some time. These physicians were evidently familiar with irrational terrors.

The housekeeper of Hippothous could in some way divine the progress of her illness by herself through an internal sense. Such prompting without organs or objects brings affliction, pleasure, fear, encouragement, hope or contempt.[196] Apparently an intuitive knowledge of one's own body not aided by external observation or by the physician was something which of itself determined all the feelings.

These clinical books bring the reader into direct contact with ancient patients, the more so because no theory is obtruded, nor any explanation explicitly offered. But other books, which are of Cnidian origin, laboriously describe, classify and attempt to explain the variety of diseases. They are harder to read and more technical; passing to them is like passing from Plato to Aristotle. Their bulk and their array of detail make it impossible to write of them except in general terms. Unlike the *Epidemics*, which from time to time mention persons and places, they are an attempt at pathology proper; their attitude to disease approaches the modern ontological theory in which diseases are treated as if they were entities in themselves. But instead of the host of microbes and viruses which go far to justify that modern attitude, the ancient pathologists had little more than the familiar humours and traditional doctrines of their imbalance. These books are also therapeutic, unlike most of *Epidemics* and *Prognostic*, so that descriptions of diseases are supplemented with lists of suitable foods, drinks and treatments, along with herbal remedies drawn from limited resources but applied in variations. In these and some other books pathology and therapy are so closely linked that some pathological notions will be mentioned under therapy.

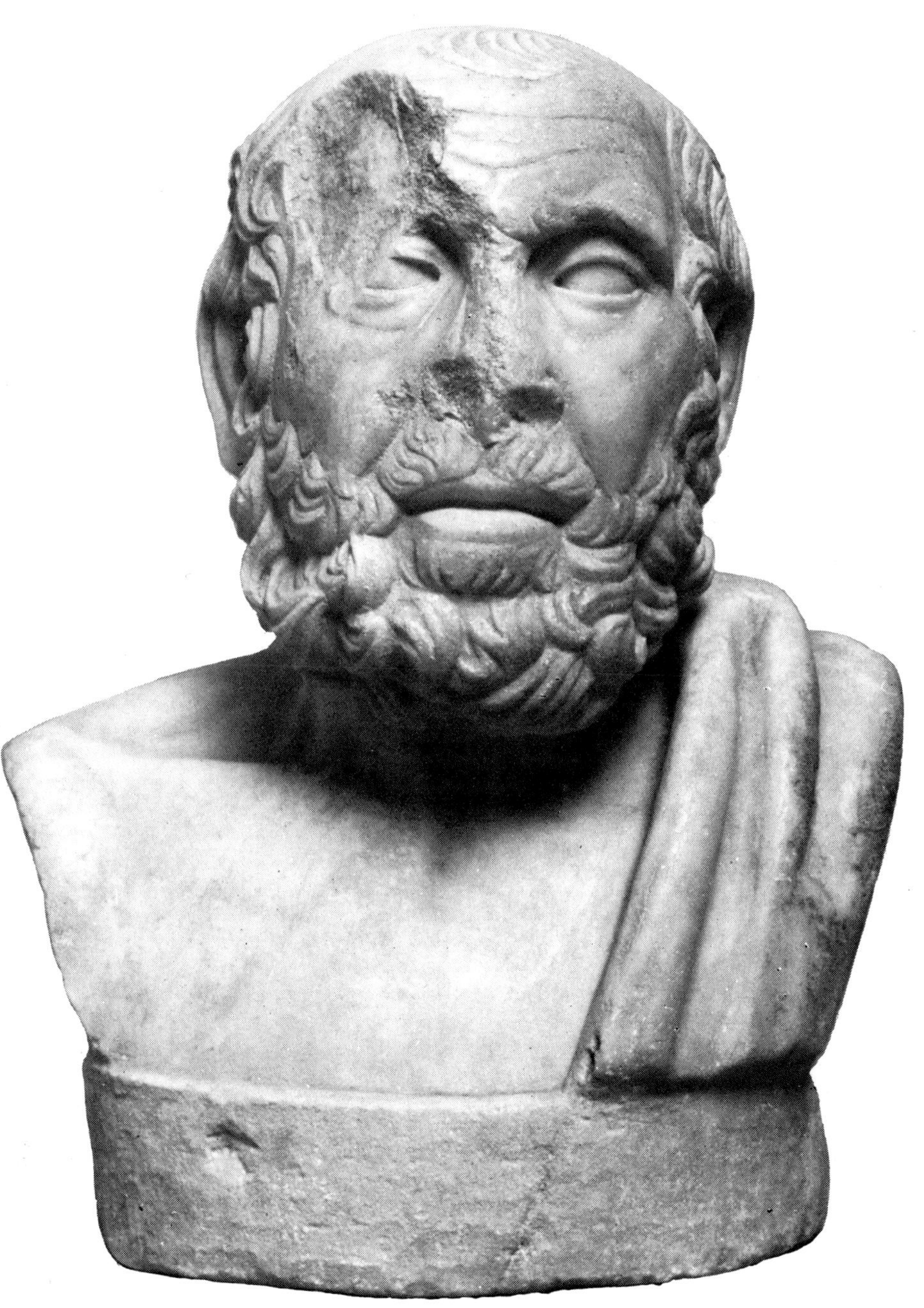

1 A Roman copy of an Hellenistic bust of Hippocrates found in the tomb of a doctor at Ostia. Although a later copy, this is probably one of the most accurate representations of Hippocrates to survive (Ostia Museum).

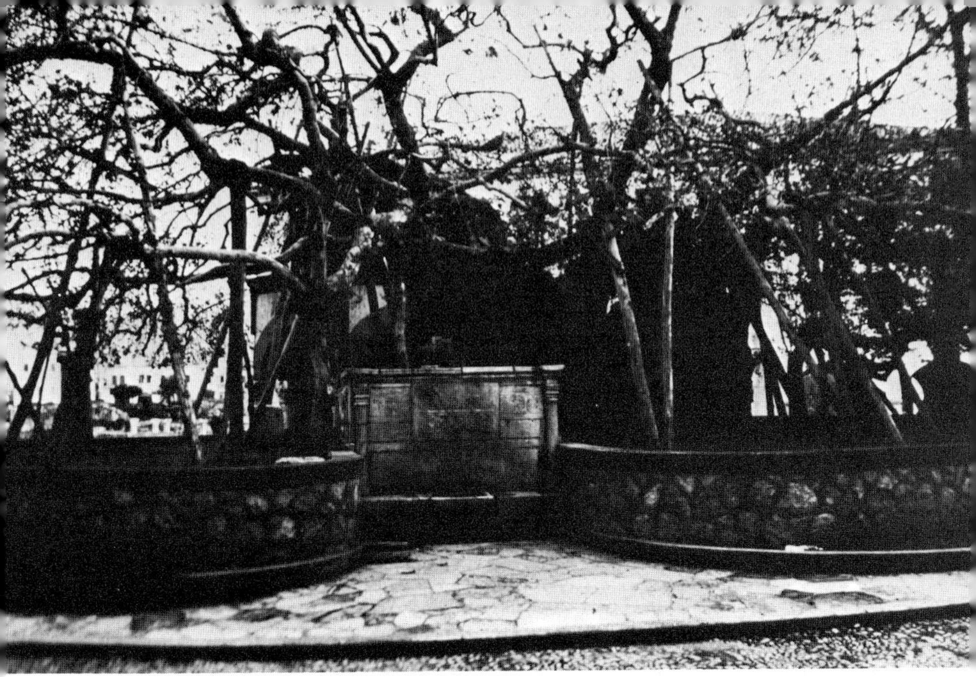

2 The island of Cos was the birthplace of Hippocrates, but this celebrated plane tree, under which he is said to have sat and taught, is now reckoned to be no more than four or five hundred years old. It may have had predecessors on the site, among which one, much older, could have been authentic.

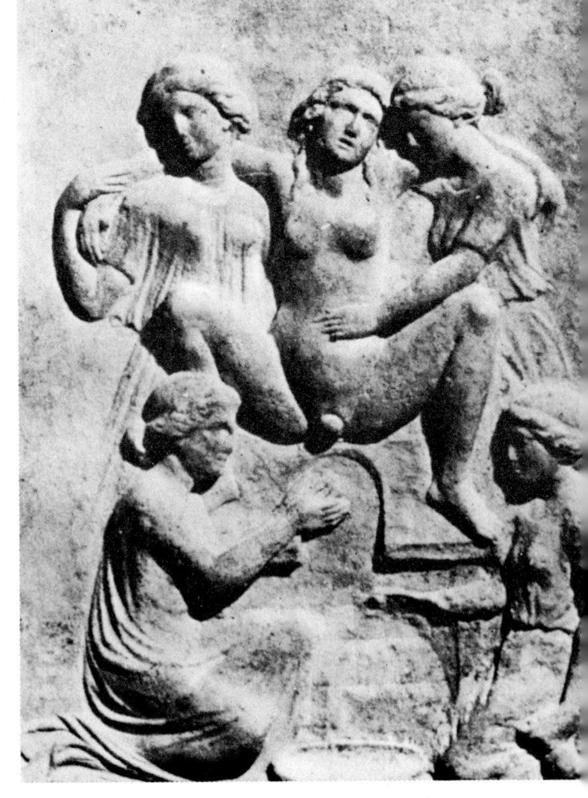

3 A fifth-century BC relief showing a birth. The mother is supported in a squatting position on a special birth chair by two attendants, who have no counterparts in the different arrangements of our own medicine. Two other attendants at the front are preparing to do the actual midwifery. They have a basin and oil ready and will catch the baby as it falls. This position of giving birth is the commonest in primitive art and society even today.

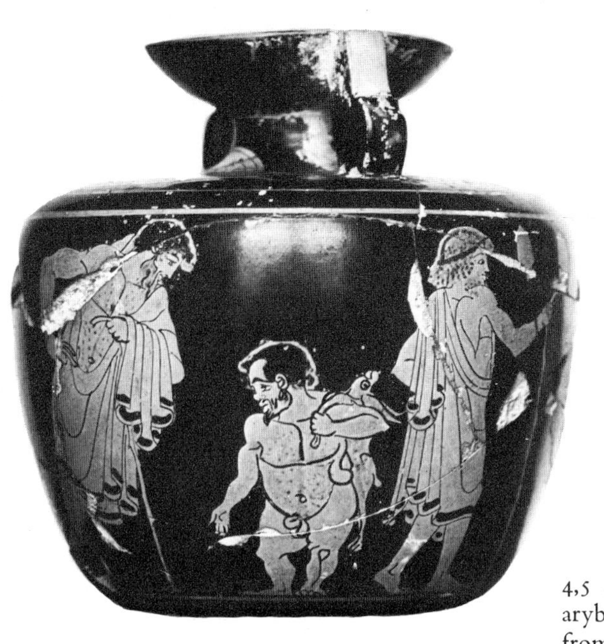

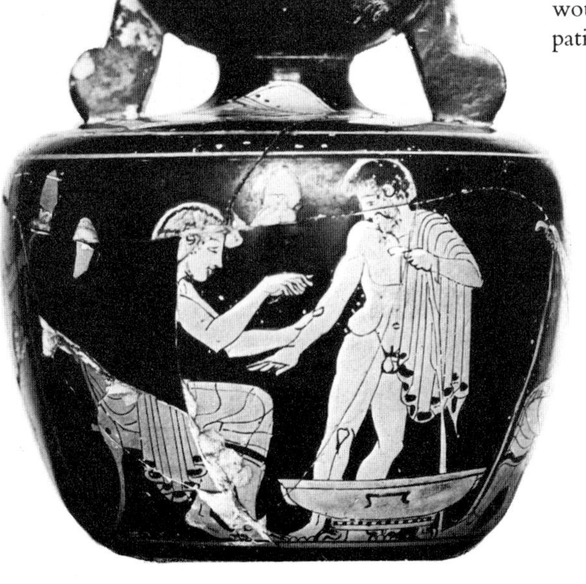

4,5 A small Attic red-figure aryballos showing scenes from a physician's surgery. *Above,* one of the queue is a powerful dwarf; *below,* the seated physician appears to be treating a wound or an injury to a patient's arm (Louvre, Paris).

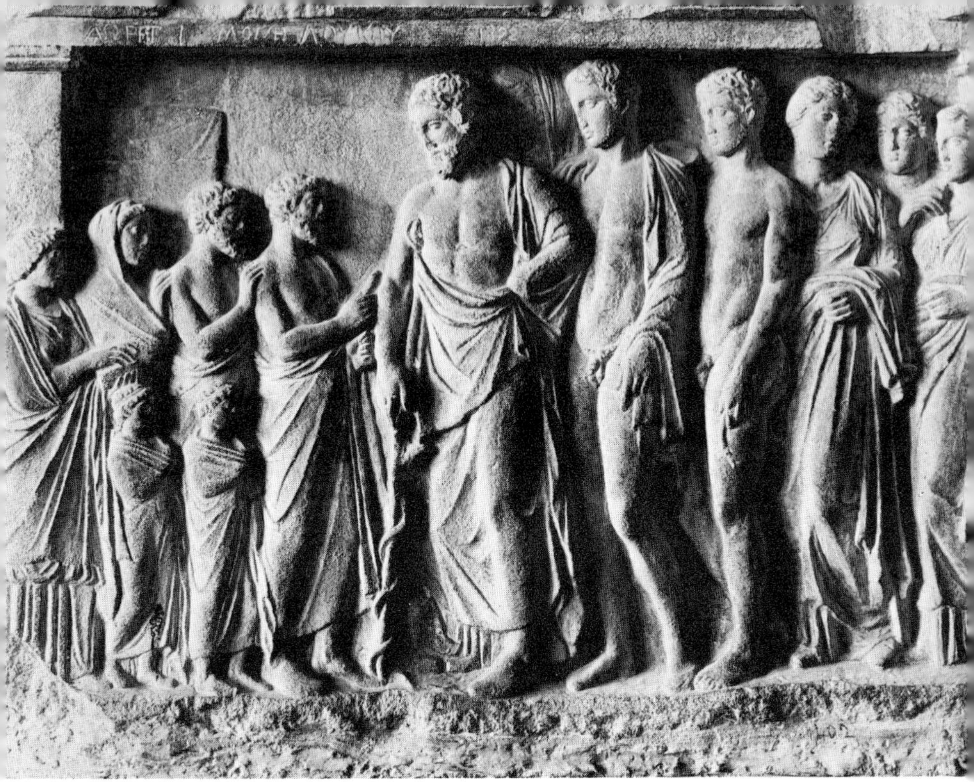

6 A votive relief dedicated to Asclepius found at Thyrea in Argolis. The shorter figures on the left are human devotees; the taller figures on the right are Asclepius and his attendant divinities, Hygieia, scarcely visible, Machaon, Podalirius, Aceso and Panacea (National Museum, Athens).

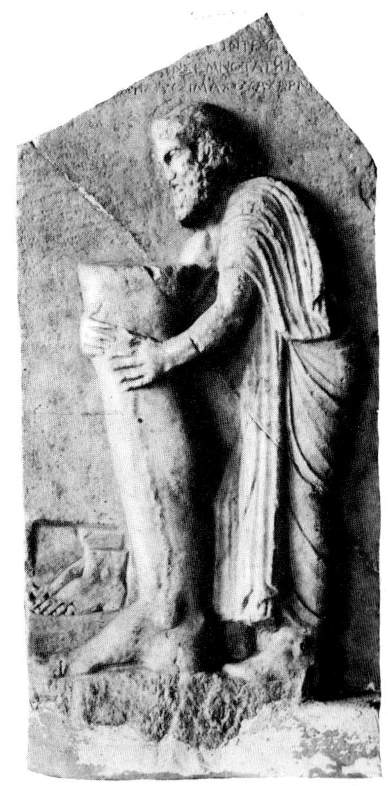

7 A votive relief dedicated to Asclepius. The dedicator presents a large ex-voto leg, but notice also the pair of feet shown in front of it. Possibly the ailment concerned was varicose veins, since a vein is shown in unusually high relief on the leg. Such reliefs served one of two purposes, either as a thank offering for a cure effected or as an entreaty for a cure from the god.

The classification of diseases is by symptoms, which are described in more detail than is found in Coan books. Varieties are distinguished for many well-known diseases that have names. Thus *Diseases* I gives five kinds of empyema, *Diseases* II five kinds of phthisis in the lungs, and *Internal Affections* (Περὶ τῶν ἐντὸς παθῶν) three kinds of phthisis, four kinds of nephritis, three kinds of leucophlegmasia, four kinds of dropsy, three kinds of hepatitis, four diseases of the spleen, four kinds of jaundice and three kinds of tetanus.[197] For explanation these writers could assume some variation in each morbid humour, but this would be the nearest approach to our conception of various microbes which might attack the same organ with similar but not identical effects. For them, differential diagnosis could very seldom be adequately based. Sometimes their humoral pathology could run parallel to ours, as with tuberculosis. Ancient writers mostly noticed only the consumption of the lungs, but if they saw similar symptoms anywhere else they could in their terms say that the peccant humour had reached other organs. A flow of morbid humours from the main site of damage was often regarded as beneficial, for it would strike a stronger or a less important part of the body and might even be drained away by the physician if it appeared as pus or in a swelling. In all Hippocratic medicine such a flow was called an *apostasis*, which in English is sometimes translated as 'abscession'. The practice of bleeding must also be seen against this background. But such a disease as cancer, for example, was hard to fit into the humoral framework.

At the beginning of *Diseases* I some necessary topics are raised on which every physician called in should have his answer ready: what is the origin of all men's illnesses; what necessities determine whether they shall be long or short, mortal or not mortal, and whether some parts of the body shall be disabled or not; what illnesses, when once they have begun, leave it doubtful whether their issue will be good or bad; what diseases will change into what others; what actions of physicians in treatment are fortunate or not, what good or evil happens to patients; what is said or done by the physician to the patient on a basis of mere conjecture, and what is said and done within medicine with precise knowledge; what is right and what is wrong; what is the beginning, middle, and end.[198] After this rhetorical preamble, some very ordinary answers are suggested.

All diseases have their internal cause in bile or phlegm, and external causes in exhaustion, wounds, stifling heat, freezing cold, parching dryness or soaking moisture. Bile and phlegm belong congenitally to the body and are always there in varying amounts, taking effect in illness by excess of heat or cold. In wounds the inevitable effect is lameness when great tendons or the heads of muscles are injured, especially in the thighs. Death results from wounds in the brain, spinal marrow, liver, diaphragm, bladder, in a haemorrhaged vein or in the heart. Other wounds are not fatal. Among diseases these can be fatal: phthisis, dropsy *anasarka*, pneumonia in pregnancy, ardent fever, phrenitis, pleurisy, angina, swollen uvula, hepatitis, swollen spleen, dysentery and, in a woman, loss of blood. The following are not mortal, unless there are complications: fluxes to the lower body causing swellings (κέδματα), melancholia or excess of dark bile, gout, coxalgia, tenesmus, quartan fever, stranguria, ophthalmia, lepra or psoriasis, scurvy, arthritis. But these last often leave permanent lesions, such as paralysis of the hands and feet, loss of voice, paraplegia due to black bile, limping as a result of coxalgia, loss of sight and hearing due to local descents of phlegm. Long-lasting diseases are phthisis, dysentery, gout, swellings from downward fluxes, leucophlegmasia, coxalgia, stranguria, nephritis in the old, fluxes of blood in women, haemorrhoids and fistulae. Crisis comes quickly in ardent fever, phrenitis, pneumonia, angina, swollen uvula and pleurisy. Pleurisy can change into ardent fever, tenesmus into dysentery, dysentery into lientery, lientery into dropsy, leucophlegmasia into dropsy, pneumonia and pleurisy into empyema.[199]

This classification is quite useful, and it does take note of complications, as we now call them. As we turn through the many pages of the other books of *Diseases*, of *Internal Affections* and of the introductory handbook *Affections* (Περὶ παθῶν), we find much clinical description somewhat in the same terms as in *Epidemics*, except that it is general and not arranged according to days, for these descriptions are not reports of individual cases.

But we find no causal agents mentioned except bile and phlegm, which are obviously made to do too much; nor are specific reasons offered, apart from those to do with their site, for the differences between one disease and another, not to speak of the varieties distinguished within each disease. Thus there was little advance in aetiology either then or for many centuries to come. The attitude towards disease was rational, but the empirical means to further understanding was absent, as we have said more than once, when neither cellular structure within the body, nor the microbes that invaded it could be seen or studied. One writer makes a good point when he distinguishes three main epochs in therapy: the first, when disease was ascribed to invading demons, the second when it was thought to arise from a lack of balance among the humours, and the third when new invaders of the body were discovered in the form of microbes and viruses.[200] Incantations or other forms of magic were used against the demons; bleeding, purging, emetics and diet were intended to remedy the imbalance among the humours; and now antiseptics and antibiotics are employed against the hostile parasites that are seen to penetrate the body. On the assumptions of its age, each one of these methods has its justification.

REGIMEN AND THERAPY

Though they understood so little of the causes of disease, the Hippocratics had a good notion of the treatment of patients in such matters as rest and comfort, washing and warming, feeding with slops and drinks to keep up the strength, and on the psychological side, too, of the sympathy and encouragement needed to keep up trust and hope. They also had a positive tradition of regimen for maintaining health when there had not yet been disease, as well as for restoring health in convalescence. With their ideas of regimen belong also their notions of hygiene or public health. Of the books dealing with regimen one concerns regimen in general, one regimen in health, and one regimen in acute diseases, and remarks on these subjects are scattered throughout the Corpus. Since the notion of regimen was so comprehensive, it will be convenient to begin with general principles and then to pass through regimen in health to regimen in sickness, returning in this way to sickness and its treatment.

In most cultures medicine was and is considered by most people negatively, as a technique for handling sickness or injury. A subject is taught in our own time called preventive medicine, but, though prevention is better than cure, even this is negative. Among the Greeks the conception of positive health was current. Those who had the means and the leisure applied themselves to maintaining positive health, which they often conceived aesthetically, and to this end put themselves into the hands of trainers, who subjected them to regimen. Training for war and for athletic competitions was of course well known among them, but these again are limited ends, while health was an excellence in its own right, the physical counterpart and condition of mental cultivation. This is a commonplace among Classical scholars or educators, who have often harped upon it to a tiresome degree, and we need say no more of it. But the details of regimen practised for health were an important part of Greek medicine, as the Hippocratics and other authors testify.

Regimen (*Περὶ διαίτης*) I requires a knowledge of man's primary constitution and of the powers of various foods, both those natural to them and those resulting from human skill.[201] This is the same doctrine that appears in *Ancient Medicine*. But eating alone is not enough for health. There must also be exercise, of which the effects must likewise be known. The combination of these two things makes regimen, when proper attention is given to the season of the year, the changes of the winds, the age of the individual and the situation of his home. If there is any deficiency either in food or exercise the body will fall sick. The author claims for himself that he can watch disease gathering gradually before it reveals itself. All animals, including man, are composed of fire and water, which must be kept in balance by regimen – fire being the principle of movement and water of nourishment. The two opposites are conceived in the style of pre-Socratic nature philosophy.[202] The whole passage shows the influence of Heraclitus in its paradoxical style and its argument that the tension of opposites sustains the universe as well as its creatures. Water and fire seem to symbolize the processes of metabolism which later medicine has called anabolic and catabolic, those which store and those which expend energy, as well as the differences between temperaments that we call calm and energetic.

Among cereals barley is cooling and drying, and so is the pottage called *kykeon*, made of barley with wine and milk, the wine adding heat; wheat is stronger and more nourishing. Food from meats boiled or fried with honey and oil is heating and windy. Spelts are lighter and more laxative. Beans are astringent and flatulent, peas less windy and more laxative. Millet, groats and husks are dry and binding, and with figs afford nourishment for physical work. Other plants are noted for their effects, healing, cooling, drying, moistening, binding or laxative. So too beef is strong and binding, goats' flesh is lighter, pork is strengthening and passes well by stool, while young pigs' flesh is hot and deranges the belly. Asses' flesh, dogs' flesh, puppies' flesh, venison, hare and hedgehog also figure in the diet. Birds are mostly drying. Fish from the sea are dry and light, except that feeders in muddy places such as mullet and eel are heavier on the stomach, and fish from rivers and ponds heavier still. Eggs and cheese are strong and nourishing. Wines are in various degrees hot and dry, but some heat without drying. A long list of vegetables follows with their effects classified in the same way, and another of fruits.[203]

Baths in fresh water moisten and cool; salt baths warm and dry; hot baths taken on an empty stomach reduce and cool; taken after a meal they warm and moisten. Cold baths dry the body and so does total abstinence from bathing. Oiling warms, moistens and softens; sun and fire dry; sweats dry and reduce, sexual intercourse reduces, moistens and warms. Vomiting reduces but does not dry, and relaxes constipated bowels. Sleep on an empty stomach reduces and cools, but after a meal warms and moistens. Want of sleep after a meal prevents the food from dissolving.[204]

Among exercises, some are called natural and others violent. Natural exercises without any violence are those of sight, hearing, voice and thought: even thought warms and dries a man and makes the flesh thin. Exercise of the voice moves the soul and makes it warm and dry. These we recognize nowadays as outputs of nervous energy, and it is quite correct to see them as using nourishment. Physical exercises are walking, running and wrestling, all of which are said to have elements of violence. Running on the double track heats and dissolves the flesh and digests the food. This kind of running makes the body slower and more gross than running on a circular track, but it is more beneficial to big eaters and in winter rather than summer. Running in a cloak heats the body more rapidly; it benefits those who have dry bodies, those who wish to reduce an excess of flesh and those who are approaching old age and are cold. The double course run with the body exposed dissolves the flesh less, making it less flabby, but reduces the body more; the exertions of it draw out the moisture from the flesh, apparently for the benefit of the inner parts of the soul. This may refer to mental strain, as the double course was the most strenuous of the foot races. Running in a circle dissolves the flesh least by sweat, but reduces the belly by rapid respiration.[205]

In persons of dry flesh jerky swinging of the arms causes sprains. Sparring and raising the body stimulate body and soul and empty the body of breath. Wrestling and massage harden the body, and are best done in winter with oil, which keeps the heat in the body, and in summer with dust, which cools it. The pains of fatigue are suffered most by untrained people. Moisture remaining in the body can even cause fever. The pains must be reduced by vapour baths, and hot baths and gentle walks. Sometimes vomiting is beneficial.[206]

These and more prescriptions in the four books of *Regimen* would take up the whole time of the person submitting to them, for they would need to be kept up without interruption. They could not be combined with regular work as we understand it.

Regimen in Health (Περὶ διαίτης ὑγιεινῆς) is much shorter. Special attention is given to the seasons. Laymen, that is those who are not professional athletes, should in winter drink as little as possible, confining themselves to unwatered wine, and eat bread and roast meat with very few vegetables. In spring, drink should be increased and diluted, food should be softer and less, with barley cake instead of bread, meat should be less and boiled instead of roasted, and vegetables should be raw or boiled. In summer the barley cake should be soft, the drink diluted and copious and all the meats boiled, to make the body cold and soft. In autumn food should be more abundant again and drier, and drinks smaller and less diluted.[207]

Special physiques need special diets beyond this. Those who are fleshy, soft and red should follow a dry regimen for most of the year to counteract their natural moistness. Those who are lean and sinewy, whether ruddy or dark, should use a moist regimen most of the time. Young people, who are naturally dry, should choose a softer and moister regimen. Older people should have a dry diet most of the time for their moist, soft and cold bodies.[208]

Walking should be rapid in winter and slow in summer, except under a burning heat. Fleshy people should walk faster, thin people slower. Bathing should be frequent in summer, less in winter, and the lean should bathe more than the fleshy. In winter cloaks should be unoiled, in summer soaked in oil – this would make them cooler. Fat people wishing to grow thin should always take exertion on an empty stomach; they should take their food while they are panting and before they are cooled. Their meat should be rich so that they will be satisfied with a minimum, and they should have only one square meal a day. Thin people wishing to be fat should do the opposite of these things, particularly avoiding exertion on an empty stomach.[209]

Emetics should be used for emptying the body during the six winter months, to rid it of phlegm above the diaphragm. In hot weather clysters should be used to remove bilious matter from the lower body. Fat people should have salty and thin clysters, lean, dry people greasy and thick ones made with milk. Fat men should take their emetics on an empty stomach, or after running or walking quickly: these should be made of hyssop, water, vinegar and salt. Thinner people should take them after food, and also after drinking dry, sweet and finally acid wines.[210]

Athletes, on the other hand, run a serious risk of diarrhoea in training. When they have it they must reduce their training by one third, and their food by one half. They should mostly have meals of baked bread broken into wine, and that once a day, until their digestions recover strength. Those who have this diarrhoea are mostly of dense flesh and their constitutions produce sudden changes for better or worse.[211] The greater liability of athletes to some illnesses during training is still well known to us.

These instructions on regimen combine some points of practical use with constant *a priori* reasoning drawn from the nature philosophers, which in that age was readily accepted as scientific.

Regimen in Acute Diseases (*Περὶ διαίτης ὀξέων*) is one of the best Cnidian books. In itself it is not long, but its *Appendix*, surely of later date, is much longer and fuller, with directions on various kinds of treatment. *Regimen in Acute Diseases* has some remarks on regimen in health, and also, with its *Appendix*, much to say on therapy, for in sickness regimen and therapy cannot be kept apart. But some of these remarks are better included under therapy, especially those in the *Appendix*.

The acute diseases actually described in this book mostly have their sites above the diaphragm and principally affect respiration. There is mention of pleurisy, pneumonia, phrenitis and ardent fever, of which the last two may be forms of malaria. The directions on regimen are concerned chiefly with food and drink, and less with emetics and purges or other things which could be called medicine. Baths are another feature, and also fomentations, but these belong rather to therapy. The writer complains that earlier Cnidian writers, who recommended purges, emetics and milk, did not pay enough attention to regimen for the sick.

For keeping up the patient's strength, barley gruel was the main food; sometimes unstrained, at other times strained so as to become mere juice. Then as later much invalid diet necessarily consisted of slops which would not overload the digestion. Among drinks hydromel (μελίκρητον), a mixture of honey and water, and oxymel (ὀξύμελι), a mixture of honey and vinegar, were administered hot or cold, and various wines. The names are easy to learn, says the writer, so that instructed laymen think that physicians, good or bad, prescribe the same things. In giving barley gruel some physicians think that it should be unstrained throughout the illness, while others consider that the patient should not swallow a grain of barley and strain the gruel through a cloth. Some will give no gruel or juice before the seventh day, and some at no time before the crisis. These differences make many people compare physicians to augurs, who will say that the flight of a bird on the left is a good omen, but the same bird on the right is a bad one.[212]

Barley gruel is to be preferred to other cereal foods because its gluten is smooth, consistent, soothing, lubricant, soft, thirst-quenching and easy to evacuate; it is not astringent, does not cause rumbling and does not swell in the bowels, for in boiling it has reached its utmost bulk.[213] Those who feed on gruel in acute diseases should not fast, but should take it without intermission except for a purge or an enema, and should have it as often as they have their meals in health. In a dry disease the ration should not be increased, but hydromel or wine should be taken before it. If on the other hand the mouth is moist and sputum from the lungs is as it should be, the quantity of gruel should be increased. The more the bowels are purged, the more this quantity should be increased until the crisis. Unstrained gruel administered from the outset is more suitable in the intervals of purging than any other diet.[214]

Gruel should be made from the finest barley, and boiled as well as possible, particularly if only the juice is to be used. The administration must be carefully timed, or great harm will follow. If food is confined in the bowels and gruel is given without first emptying them, it will greatly increase existing pain, or cause pain if there was none; it will also make respiration more rapid, drying the lungs and causing discomfort in the diaphragm and below. If pain in the side continues and sputum has not been brought up but is viscid and made more so by the rapid breathing that it causes, and if neither purging nor venesection has been carried out, the patient will quickly die. The rules for giving pure juice are much the same.[215]

If the fever begins soon after a meal and the bowels have not yet been emptied, give for the time being only oxymel, warm in winter and cold in summer. If there is great thirst give hydromel and water. Immediately after the patient has swallowed the purge and it has acted, give the patient gruel or juice. Again, at the beginning do not starve him for two or three days or more before giving gruel and drink. Never make sudden changes of regimen in disease or in health.[216]

Sometimes patients are changed from fasting to gruel exactly when the opposite should have been done, as when an exacerbation comes during a diet of gruel. Crude matters may then be drawn from the head and bilious matters from the chest. The patient suffers from sleeplessness, and the unconcocted matters of the disease make him depressed, peevish and delirious; his eyes suffer from flashes of light, his ears are full of noise, his extremities are chilled, his urine is unconcocted and his sputum thin and salty. He has sweats about the neck, and the ascent of his breath is interrupted, being either rapid or very deep. His eyebrows frown and he has distressing faints; he throws the clothes off his chest, trembles in the hands and sometimes his lower lip shakes. These are the initial symptoms of violent delirium, and usually he dies.[217] Among these symptoms the disturbed breathing may be an early mention of the Cheyne-Stokes respiration of modern medicine.

Sometimes more food and drink are wrongly given when the patient is weak with the pain and sharpness of the disease. But sometimes the physician fails to see that weakness is due to lack of nourishment. In that case another physician who does see this may help the patient greatly, so that to the public he appears to be raised from the dead. This mistake brings the first physician into contempt. From rest, the body should be gradually accustomed to more exertion, not suddenly be made to undergo fatigue; this is true of every part of it, including the bowels, which suffer when there is a change from strict fasting to gruel diet.[218]

There are criteria for deciding when sweet, vinous, white or dark wine should be administered. Sweet wine causes less heaviness in the head than vinous, goes to the brain less and evacuates more, but swells the spleen and liver. It makes the bilious thirsty and causes flatulence in the upper intestine, but does not disagree proportionately with the lower intestine. The flatulence from sweet wine persists in the hypochondrium. It is more expectorant than vinous white wine, but less diuretic and laxative.[219]

A pale white wine and an astringent dark wine may be used in acute diseases if there is no heaviness in the head, no affection of the brain, no checking of sputum and no stopping of urine, and if the bowels are loose. If it is diluted it will do less harm to the upper parts and the bladder; if it is less diluted it will be better for the bowels.[220]

Hydromel taken throughout is less suited to the bilious and large of belly. It causes less thirst than sweet wine, softens the lungs and is mildly expectorant and diuretic. It is most effective in bringing up sputum when it is diluted with water. Taken neat it will provoke frothy stools in the bilious, causing distress and tossing and ulceration of the intestines and seat. It is nutritive unless it deranges the digestion, but less nutritive than neat wine or neat honey. If it is drunk after barley gruel it will cause flatulence and trouble in the bowels, but before the gruel it does no harm. Boiled hydromel is bright and transparent but less nutritious.[221]

Oxymel brings up sputum and eases respiration. When it is acid it has great effect, unless it makes the sputum viscid, as it may in those who have not the strength to cough. So it must not be given unless there is hope of recovery, and then it should be taken tepid and in small doses. Slightly acid oxymel moistens the mouth, brings up sputum and quenches thirst. It may prevent flatulence from passing out of the lower intestines and make them too moist, but that is its only ill effect. If it is drunk alone without gruel, any oxymel may roughen the intestines, which suffer more since in this case the patient is fasting. In large quantity it should have as little vinegar in it as possible. The acidity of the vinegar dissolves bitter bile, but ferments black bile.[222]

Water has little advantage as a drink in fever, for it does not quench thirst, increases bile, and if drunk during a fast enlarges the spleen and liver. It causes gurgling and does not descend, so that it does not increase faeces. It is particularly harmful if it is drunk when the feet are cold.[223]

The bath is beneficial to many patients, sometimes when used continually, sometimes at intervals. To be carried out well, it must be given in a covered place free from smoke with abundant water. Rubbing with liquid soap (of powder and olive oil) should be done only if the soap is warm and more abundant than usual.

The passage to the basin should be short and the basin easy for stepping in and stepping out. The bather should be quiet, silent and passive. Sponges should be used instead of a scraper, and the body should be anointed before it is quite dry. The head should be sponged as nearly dry as possible. The bath should not be given soon after gruel or drink, nor should these follow it too soon. The patient's normal habits of bathing are very important. Bathing suits pneumonia rather than ardent fevers, for it soothes the pain in the chest, brings up sputum, eases respiration and removes heaviness in the head. Do not bathe those with loose or constipated bowels, or those who are liable to nausea, vomiting, or bleeding from the nose. Those who are fit to take unstrained gruel are more capable of bathing than those who take only juice.[224]

Regimen of rather this kind for fever has persisted until a time within living memory. The marked change in our own generation has been made by the use of antibiotics.

We come now to therapy, that is, to more active interference in the course of an illness than change of diet, purging or induced vomiting. In therapy the Hippocratics were cautious and gentle, as also mostly in such surgery as they undertook. Some well-known pronouncements of theirs on the subject may be quoted by way of introduction.

First, there was always for the Hippocratics a fundamental question: to treat or not to treat? So in *The Art* physicians are defended for refusing to undertake desperate cases where the illness is too strong for medicine, lest they become a laughing-stock.[225] Again, in *Diseases* I it is said that things which can be done should be conceived and mentioned, and done when it is necessary, but that things which cannot be done should not be conceived, mentioned or done.[226] These passages are rhetorical, but they need not be untrue of practice. In ancient times sedatives or drugs such as morphine were not at the physician's disposal, though now their use can be called treatment, even if it merely relieves pain without any effect on the disease. The Hippocratic physicians must often have been obliged to let patients die without any mitigation of suffering.

Their aim was to do good, or at least to do no harm; this is stated in *Epidemics* I, which also lays down that the art of medicine has three factors, the disease, the patient and the physician, who is the servant of the art, and that the patient must help the physician in combating the disease.[227] In *Epidemics* VI we find the judgment that the constitutions are the healers of diseases.[228] This implies that the human physician is simply the assistant of nature which actually does the healing. In the first section of *Aphorisms* (*'Αφορισμοί*) are more such judgments. Life is short, the art long, opportunity fleeting, experiment full of pitfalls and decision difficult. The physician must not only show himself as doing his duty, but must also have the patient, the attendants, and external things ready for this.[229]

Rather more particular are the following maxims. In *Aphorisms* VII degrees of intervention are recommended as follows. Those diseases which medicine cannot cure, the knife cures; those which the knife does not cure, fire cures. Those that fire does not cure you must consider incurable.[230] *Aphorisms* I contains the warning that a restricted and rigid regimen is treacherous both in chronic diseases and in acute ones where it is not required.[231] Any extreme of restriction or repletion is perilous. In a restricted regimen the patient's mistakes are more serious than in a liberal one, and the same is true even in health. But for extreme diseases extreme strictness is most effective, and should be used while the illness is at its height. Fasting is most easily endured by old men and after them by the middle-aged; it affects youths very badly and children worst of all, especially if they are unusually lively.[232]

Intervention beyond purges and emetics was confined to such remedies as fomentations, bleeding, cautery, draining the lungs and the treatment of wounds and ulcers. Thus *Regimen in Acute Diseases* advises hot fomentations when there is pain in the side. The best fomentation is hot water in a skin or bladder, or in a vessel of bronze or earthenware. Between it and the side something soft should be applied for comfort, such as a big soft sponge dipped in hot water and squeezed out. The outer side of this must be covered to hold in the heat and steam. A poultice of barley, vetches or bran may also be used. Venesection will not end the pain unless it is one that reaches the collar-bone, but, if the vein is to be cut, do so at the elbow and draw off plenty of blood.[233]

The *Appendix* to *Regimen in Acute Diseases* has much more to say of bleeding. It recommends it in an acute illness if the patient is at his most vigorous age. When the hypochondrium is swollen, the diaphragm tense, breathing interrupted and there is orthopnoea, or when there is pain in the liver, heaviness of the spleen or violent pain above the diaphragm, bleeding is the sovereign remedy; but it must be carried out in moderation if it accompanies purging.[234] These are all measures taken for excess of phlegm. Bleeding is also good for sudden loss of speech due to overfilled veins and occurring in a healthy person without external cause. The vein on the inner side of the right arm should be opened and blood drawn out as suits the constitution and age of the patient.[235] Again when pains have become fixed in a point which draws fluxes of black bile and biting humours, the veins are irritated there, becoming dry, distended and inflamed so that the blood and *pneuma* cannot flow along their natural paths. There follow chilling, dimming of the sight, loss of speech, heaviness in the head and convulsions when the stoppage reaches the heart, the liver or the great veins. When fluxes reach surrounding places there is epilepsy or paralysis. In such cases use fomentations and immediately afterwards bleeding, while the *pneuma* and humours are still in movement. In pleurisy and pneumonia, if the pain is very acute, the bleeding must be carried on until the patient faints. Among precautions to be taken before bleeding it is recommended that the patient be made costive and kept on a low diet.[236]

Bleeding was thought to cure more conditions still: eye disease, stranguria, dysuria are mentioned in *Aphorisms*, and in *Epidemics* loss of voice without fever, orchitis, digestive disorder with violent rumbling, and lack of nourishment from food.[237] Diversionary bleeding is also a favourite theme in *Epidemics* V. One Eudemus is reported to have had much pain in the right buttock, in the groin and on the inner side of the thigh. A great quantity of thick dark blood was drawn off from his ankle, a distant point, and he swallowed a purge. Then he was cauterized on the buttock with many scars, and pus ran out. A few days later he died, as much from the size and number of his wounds as from exhaustion. The writer thinks that if one large incision had been made to draw out the pus, and perhaps one other, at the right time, the patient would have recovered.[238] There are many more Greek references to bleeding. In Europe it remained in favour till the early years of the nineteenth century.

Cautery was quite as common as bleeding, to judge by the many references – too many, indeed, to quote in detail. The commonest use of all was to open and drain empyema from the lungs. *Prognostic* warns that when an empyema is opened by cautery or incision the patient survives if the pus is clean, white and has not a bad smell, but dies if it is bloody and turbid.[239] In *Aphorisms* VI is another warning, that if incision or cautery is practised and the pus or water is drained all at once the patient dies.[240] Cautery for empyema is mentioned likewise in *Aphorisms* VII, *Epidemics* IV and *Coan Prognoses* (*Κωακαὶ προγνώσεις*) II.[241] In *Joints* (*Περὶ ἄρθρων ἐμβολῆς*) it is recommended rather oddly to prevent a shoulder-joint that has been reduced from becoming dislocated again.[242] *Aphorisms* VII mentions it as a remedy for spontaneous dislocations of the thigh.[243] These uses of it were intended to burn away loose flesh and tighten the joints.

So also in *Airs, Waters, Places* the Scythians are said to cauterize their shoulders, arms, wrists, breasts, buttocks and groins to reduce the natural softness and moistness of their constitutions by burning away the humours.[244] A more natural use appears in *Epidemics* V, where it is advised when suppuration follows a fracture of the ribs.[245] Its main purpose is clearly either to drain by piercing a hole, or to dry and tense various parts of the body. The pain is not mentioned, not even in references to cautery of the ear in *Joints* or to cautery of the veins around the eye in *Places in Man*.[246]

The procedure for draining the lungs, whether cautery or incision was used, is described in *Diseases* II under abscess of the lung and empyema resulting from pneumonia. Before these operations are attempted, various concoctions of fruit juice, honey, salt, grease, flower juices and vinegar are to be poured warm down the windpipe while the patient's tongue is pulled outward, or a balsam of frankincense, wine, mild and other substances is to be inhaled through a tube, and followed by more infusions; the infusions, as described, seem calculated to choke the patient if they really flowed down his windpipe. If these methods fail to bring out the pus, the patient must be washed in hot water and seated on a firm chair while his arms are held. By shaking his shoulders and by careful auscultation the place where the râle is most clearly heard will be determined. One should try to make the incision on the left side where it is less dangerous. Sometimes there is too much pus for auscultation. Then you will make the incision as low as possible on the side where the swelling and pain are greatest, and behind the swelling. The cut must be made between the ribs with a convex knife in the outer skin, and then a pointed knife must be wrapped in linen with its tip left bare for the distance of a thumbnail and driven into the wound. When you have drawn off as much pus as seems right, insert a plug of unbleached lint with a thread attached. Draw off the pus once a day. On the tenth day, when you have drawn it all off, put in a linen plug. Then inject warm wine and oil through a pipe so that the lung, which has become accustomed to being bathed in pus, will not dry too quickly. Take out the morning's injection in the evening, and the evening's in the morning. When the pus is as thin as water, viscous to the touch and scanty, put in a tube of hollow tin. When the interior is completely dry, cut off part of the tube little by little and cicatrize the wound until you withdraw the tube altogether. If the pus has been white and clear throughout there will be a cure, but if it is yellow and fetid the patient will die when it is all drained.[247]

This kind of treatment was applied to various sorts of wound and to fistulae, but not to wounds in the head nor incisions in the ear. Ulcers were sometimes difficult to treat. *Epidemics* VI reports that a man who had a rodent ulcer high on the side of his head benefited at first from treatment with burned alum, but had another vent elsewhere because the bone was on the point of exfoliation. It did exfoliate on the sixtieth day.[248] In *Places in Man* the treatment advised for a larger and worse ulcer, which spreads as its discharge infects the surrounding flesh, is to anoint the ulcer itself with moistening remedies, which will allow the discharge to flow out without spreading through the raw flesh. The still unharmed flesh must be compacted with cooling drugs, which should be applied all round the ulcer. It is not stated what the drugs are.[249]

In *Ulcers* (*Περὶ ἑλκῶν*), which covers both ulcers and some wounds, various drugs are prescribed for the treatment of particular lesions. From this book and some others a Hippocratic pharmacopoeia could be put together, though it would not be systematic or comprehensive. In several places a book called *Pharmakitis* is mentioned which may have been comprehensive, but it is lost.[250] But even the drugs which are mentioned are too numerous to be listed in this book. It must suffice to reproduce one or two lists of drugs as they are prescribed for definite conditions. These vegetable or mineral remedies were supplied by traditional traders or collectors to the physicians, who used them for their known effects with little or no explanatory theory.

Thus in *Ulcers* it is laid down that wounds must be kept as dry as possible, for that state is nearest to the healthy state, and the moist state to the diseased. This is a general view in ancient medicine and nature philosophy. The only moistening should be with wine – regarded in ancient medicine as a disinfectant. An exception is made for lesions in joints, no doubt because drying would make them hard to bend or stretch. While a wound or ulcer is under treatment food and drink should be reduced to a minimum; this is particularly necessary with recent wounds, and with all that may become inflamed. Suppuration must be hastened as much as possible, and the wound then dried by a remedy which is not irritant. This is particularly required for contused wounds to keep them from festering. For the same purpose, a quantity of blood must be drawn from a wound, and also from chronic ulcers to reduce swelling. A sponge should be applied, and leaves above it. Oil should not be used until the place is nearly healed. Wounds in the head, belly and joints, and those which may become gangrenous, as well as rodent and creeping ulcers, should be drained downwards.[251]

When the draining, drying and cleaning are finished it is time to apply remedies. Swollen and inflamed wounds should be covered with a plaster made of mullein, raw clover leaves, boiled rock plant and hulwort, which all have a further cleansing effect.[252] So have the leaves of fig trees, olive trees, and horehound, which should be boiled, as should agnus castus and pomegranate leaves.[253] Other plants should be applied raw: mallow, rue and organy should be pounded with wine and roasted flax seed.[254] To prevent erysipelas occurring on wounds woad should be used raw with flax seed, or moistened flax seed with the juice of houndsberry or woad.[255] If after cleaning the wound tries to inflame the neighbouring parts, lentils pounded and cooked with wine and oil should be applied as a plaster and a bandage put over this, or boiled caper pounded very small and covered in a linen bandage soaked in wine and oil. To bring together the edges of a wound, caper leaves, lentils and nose-smart should be mixed with wine and pounded flax seed.[256] Flax seed with raw agnus castus and Melian alum soaked in vinegar may also be applied. These herbal remedies must have taken generations to discover and their use must extend far back into the primitive past.

Beside vegetable remedies, minerals of various kinds are advised for drying and disinfecting ulcers and wounds. They were reduced to powders and sprinkled on; such were Egyptian and Melian alum as astringents or styptics, also oxides of copper, called by such names as 'Cyprian dust' and 'flowers of copper'. There were also oxide of lead, called *lithargyros* or 'flower of silver' because of its lustre, and sulphate of lead, called *molybdaina*.[257] The use of metallic oxides or sulphates seems odd, but they are forerunners of the powders we apply to wounds and sores.

Herbs and minerals of these kinds were used particularly for staunching the flow of blood when this was desired, and to dry up suppuration. Some of them also appear among preparations for the treatment of fistulae and of bleeding piles in the books concerned with these maladies.

Other treatments, some of which amount to minor operations, are dealt with in *Diseases* II. Among them a disorder is mentioned more than once in which the blood vessels of the head, spewing back the blood which should pass through them, heat the head and cause a violent fever, with pain in the temples, bregma and occiput. The ears sing and are full of wind; the patient hears nothing and tosses continually with pain until he dies, usually on the fifth or sixth day unless treated. In such a case his head should be heated with fomentations until water erupts through his ears and nostrils. Some scholars have called the disease apoplexy, which was attributed to blocking of the vessels by phlegm. The treatment was intended to dissipate the phlegm by further heat. A similar disease could be treated by incising the bregma and drawing off blood there.[258]

A disease called *kynanche*, which usually means quinsy, was in fact evidently more serious than the name suggests.[259] It brought fever, shivering, headache, swelling under the jaws, difficulty in salivation and spitting out hard matter in small pieces. There was a râle at the bottom of the throat, and later the patient could not spit. He could not breathe lying down. Cupping glasses were to be applied to the back of his neck by the first vertebra and left for a long time. Then he was to have an inhalation of a liquid made with vinegar, soda, organy and watercress (all pounded), water and a little oil. This was to be heated on charcoal and breathed in through a hollow reed, while sponges of hot water were applied to the patient's jaws and below. A gargle of herbs was also to be taken and the throat cleaned out with a ball of soft wool on the end of a stick of myrtle. There might be a swelling on the chest, red and burning, which would be a good sign, for the phlegm would have made an *apostasis* to this spot.[260] The apparatus for inhalation recalls the kettles used for vapour in cases of bronchitis.

A similar fever was treated by inserting tubes into the throat along the jaws, so that air might be drawn into the lungs. A fumigation of hyssop was to be inhaled through the nostrils and the tubes, and the throat and tongue covered with phlegmagogues. The veins were cut under the tongue and blood was also drawn from the bend of the arm.[261]

Water on the brain, felt at the bregma and at the temples, can cause shuddering and fever, pain in the eyes, double vision, vertigo, noises in the ears, and thinning of the skin of the head so that the patient likes to have it touched. After administering emetics to draw the phlegm, clearing the nose with an errhine and purging the bowels, feed the patient well and let him take walks out of the sun and wind. If there is no improvement after some time on this treatment, cut his head open at the bregma, perforating as far as the brain, and treat the incision as you would trepanation.[262] Blood must surely have been drawn out here as well as some of the escaped cerebro-spinal fluid.

A polypus in the nose which hindered breathing could be removed in various ways. One method was simply to pull it out. Four linen threads were attached to a tight ball of sponge, with their other ends passed through an eyehole in a tapering metal rod. The rod was then thrust up the nostril into the mouth, and onward, while the uvula was pressed out of the way. The whole apparatus was then pulled out through the mouth so that the sponge dragged the polypus with it. The bleeding was then stopped with a plug of linen soaked in paste of flowers of copper and honey. The final healing was done with a leaden rod smeared with honey and pressed against the scar. The rod would need to be rather flexible. The polypus could also be cauterized with a hot iron introduced inside a tube, and the wound plugged with linen treated as before. An elongated polypus, said to be hard and to sound like a stone when it was touched, had to be removed by slitting open the nostril followed by cautery. The healing of the wound when sewn up was the same as in the other cases.[263]

Such are a few examples of active treatment including minor surgery. But these concern places or organs which could be reached from outside. Internal therapy was attempted only by the usual purges, emetics, sudorifics, sternutatories and other drugs, which were intended to draw out the humours, or to draw them from one place to another less dangerous. According to the humoral pathology there was little else to be done.

SURGERY

After medicinal therapy it is natural to turn to surgery. Hippocratic surgery was nearly always concerned with bones and their accompanying tissues; it did not operate on soft parts except in such cases as the draining of the lung, which has been noticed. The surgery recommended and carried out by the authors of the excellent surgical books has been generally admired. In the interests of completeness some of the treatments which they do not recommend but mention with great disapproval will be added here.

The most notable of the surgical books is that which in its two sections is called *Fractures* (*Περὶ ἀγμῶν*) and *Joints*, but was probably one treatise, though it has been mutilated. *Fractures* treats of the arm, the foot, the leg and thigh, and the shoulder, with a full account of dangers such as protrusion and elimination of bone, of overriding and other malformation due to lack of surgical skill, of ulceration, inflammation and dislocation, which is treated at greater length in the succeeding section. *Joints* deals with dislocation of the shoulder joint, including avulsion of the acromion and fracture of the clavicle, of the elbow, wrist, hand and fingers, lower jaw (both dislocation and fracture), nose and ear, vertebrae in scoliosis and cyphosis, hip-joint, leg-bones and ankle, fingers and toes, with observation on dangers such as gangrene in wounds. The subject is wider than dislocations in themselves, since some diseases are mentioned in this connection. In both *Fractures* and *Joints* there is the fullest description of the necessary apparatus and treatment, of bandages and splints in the first, of leverage and wooden apparatus in the second. There are warnings against mistakes in both, and condemnations of entire methods of treatment in *Joints*. Naturally the anatomy of these bones and joints is well understood.

In *Fractures*, after a lost introduction, the writer speaks of putting up a fractured forearm for bandaging. The forearm is assumed to be held out in pronation with the elbow bent. Any position with the whole arm straight, as for instance the left arm is when holding the bow in archery, is condemned as absurd and uncomfortable. The surgeon's work is easier if only one of the two bones in the forearm is broken, preferably if it is the radius, for the ulna requires stronger extension. If both bones are broken, very strong extension is required. While the bone is held in extension the broken parts at the fracture should be pressed into position with the palms, and when the arm is put up the patient should have his hand not lower than the elbow but a little higher, so that blood may not flow to the extremity. The first bandages should be short, with their heads set on the fracture to support it without much pressure; then compresses should be applied, anointed with a little cerate, and over them bandages laid crosswise to right and left alternately, and running mostly from below upwards, but sometimes the other way.

The patient should feel a moderate pressure, chiefly at the fracture, and should also feel the pressure increasing while a slight and soft swelling should appear on the hand. But on the third day the pressure should seem less and the bandage be loose. There should always be more pressure of bandaging over the fracture itself so that the serious effusions are driven away from it and not on to it as a result of pressure elsewhere. More bandages should be used each time there is a new dressing. Within three days there should be seven dressings, and at the end of that period the fractured part should be found thin and the bones more mobile and ready for adjustment. When the bones have been adjusted, splints should be applied round the limb in ligatures and the bandages made a little tighter. No more pressure should be made by the splints, which are put on simply to maintain the dressing. They should not be laid in the line of the thumb or of the little finger, but if any are so laid they should not reach the bony projections of the wrist for fear of ulceration and denuding of tendons. The splint should be left in place for more than twenty days so that the bones of the forearm can unite. Clearly they form an openwork tube about the forearm. As much as possible of the arm and wrist should be slung evenly on a soft broad scarf.[264]

A fractured humerus should first be extended in the following manner. The arm should hang downward with the elbow bent at right angles so that the muscles on it are neither bunched nor stretched. A horizontal rod suspended by a cord at each end should pass evenly under the armpit, so that the patient, who will be seated on a high stool, is almost suspended. The forearm should next be laid on leather cushions on another stool. The broken humerus, or rather its lower end, must then be forced and kept down by heavy weights or by a strong man's grip. Then it can be adjusted and bandaged. The bandaging must be repeated every third day with greater pressure, and the limb put up in splints on the seventh or ninth day. It should consolidate in forty days. Care must be taken that its naturally convex curve outward is not distorted in the setting.[265]

Surgeons and patients are warned of the intricate anatomy of the foot, with its many small bones which must be carefully pressed into place after any injury. The same care is needed as for the hand, but for a different reason, namely that the foot bears so much weight. The passage dealing with the hand in corresponding fashion is lost. Great damage can be done in leaping down from a height and landing violently on the heel, which causes extravasation, contusion, swelling and severe pain. Bandaging with one turn round the foot and the next round the back tendon compresses the wrong parts and excludes the contused heel, so that there is a risk of necrosis of the heel bone; this may become chronic, producing illness elsewhere, even acute fever.[266]

Where fractures of the thighbone or of the lower leg-bones had to be treated, great efforts were needed to extend the broken limbs in correct line so that there would be no deformity and the pieces of bone would not override one another, that is, be drawn past one another by the tendons, which are normally somewhat stretched when the bones are unbroken. Two or more strong men might be needed to maintain the extension; alternatively leather thongs might be passed round the ends, or the affected limb attached to a post or even a windlass. While the patient's body was held, or sometimes shored against a peg or pummel set in the fork of the legs, traction would be applied by pulling the limb or turning the windlasses until the broken bones were properly laid end to end, and could be pressed by the surgeon's palms into the exact position required. The surgeon practising in a large town is recommended to get a wooden apparatus in which all these forcible methods of stretching for fractures and levering for dislocations are included. There is still some disagreement among scholars on the exact working and nature of this apparatus.[267]

Among many other remarks on traction, cleansing and bandaging, one device for maintaining extension in a fracture of the leg below the knee is worth mentioning. Two large, soft, rounded circlets sewn in Egyptian leather should be made, one to fit below the knee, the other above the ankle. They should be fitted with leather thongs, single or double and short like loops. Then, four rods of cornel wood of equal length and of the thickness of a finger should be fitted at each end, into one of the leather loops at top and bottom. They must be a little longer than the distance between the circlets, so that they exert pressure on the holding loops and through them on the knee and ankle, holding these joints far enough apart to maintain the proper extension of the fractured bone. The effect would be to make a tubular truss round the leg, which would allow easy access between the rods for dressing the fracture, and would not so press at either end as to cause sores or ulcers.[268]

Joints contains a list of dislocations and instructions for their treatment by powerful leverage. It treats of dislocated and broken jaws, broken noses and fractures of the ear, which are likely to have resulted from boxing with the hard and heavy *cestus*, used where we use a soft boxing glove. But more convenient examples for a general account are dislocations of the shoulder, humerus, wrist, hand, hip and thigh.

A dislocated humerus will show its head in the armpit, for this dislocation is always downward, and the elbow will stand out further from the ribs than on the sound side of the body, while the acromion will project on the shoulder. Reduction consists in pushing up the humerus until its head is once more in contact with the very shallow socket on which it should articulate. This can sometimes be done by the patient himself if he inserts the fist of his other hand into the armpit to push up the bone, while he draws the elbow towards his chest. The practitioner can sometimes do it by putting his fingers under the armpit inside the head of the dislocated bone to force the head away from the ribs, thrusting his own head against the top of the patient's shoulder to hold it and with his knees pressing the patient's elbow to force the lower end of the humerus against the ribs. Another method is to bring the patient's forearm backwards on to the spine and in this position to press upwards on the elbow; yet another is to make the patient lie on his back with a hard ball strapped in his armpit, to pull his arm and at the same time press firmly with the heel on the ball to force back the head of the humerus. The patient's sound shoulder should be firmly held by another person to stop his body from being drawn round, and someone should press his foot against the top of the dislocated shoulder. Again, a man taller than the patient can hang the patient's arm over his own shoulder, grasp it, and thrust the point of his shoulder into the patient's armpit. He then lifts up the patient thus suspended, and shakes him while he still holds down the dislocated arm. These methods can be used without any apparatus in the palaestra.

More artificially, the patient's armpit can be forced down on to a pestle with a soft band wrapped round its top, both his arm and his body being dragged downward while the pestle's head forces up the head of the humerus. This can also be done with a rounded object set on the step of a ladder. A more powerful method is to use a piece of wood of flattish cross-section, two cubits or less in length and rounded at one end, which has a slight rim and is covered in linen. Insert the tip of the instrument in the patient's armpit as far as possible between the ribs and the head of the humerus and tie the whole arm securely to the instrument at several points. Then fasten a cross-bar firmly between two posts a little higher than the patient's armpit. Lift the arm tied to the instrument over the cross-bar so that the armpit rests on it, then press down the arm on one side of it and on the other hold down the rest of the body, which will be suspended on tiptoe and act as a weight. By this method the instrument, keeping the arm rigid, acts as a lever, with the cross-bar as fulcrum, to force up the head of the humerus. The extremities of the arm and of the instrument are moved through an arc in the action of leverage. The same effect can be achieved by using a sufficiently strong high-backed chair or the lower half of a double door in place of the cross-bar.[269] No doubt in these cases the patient would kneel instead of standing if the weight of his body were still needed.

Dislocation is commoner in thin and lightly muscled patients or in those whose flesh is humid and less dense. The shoulder should afterwards be rubbed and bandaged, and the patient should be warned to treat the joint carefully for some time. He will be unsuitable for gymnastic contests and for warfare.[270]

The wrist is said to be dislocated inwards, that is forwards, or outwards, that is backwards, but mostly inwards. If inwards, the patient cannot flex his fingers; if outwards, he cannot extend them. In reduction the fingers should be placed on a table and assistants should make extension and counter-extension. The operator with palm or heel should then press back the projecting bone downward or forward, having put some soft mass under the other bone. If the dislocation is upwards, the hand should be prone, if downwards, supine. The bones are the two bones of the forearm where they form the wrist and meet the hand. When they are dislocated either way the flexor or extensor tendons, as the case may be, are on the stretch. Treatment is conducted by means of bandages.[271]

The hand can be completely dislocated inwards, outwards, or to either side, but the inward dislocation is commonest. Sometimes the epiphysis is displaced (that is, the lower end of the radius is fractured), and sometimes one of the bones is separated. In these cases strong extension is necessary. The projecting part must be pressed back with counter-pressure on the other side at the same time. The hand or the heel should be used and the operation performed on a table. Afterwards there must be bandaging of the hand and forearm, and splints must be applied which reach the fingers; these should be changed more frequently than with fractures. Dislocation of the finger-joint must be reduced by extending in a direct line and pressing back the projecting part, with counter-pressure on the opposite side. Treatment should be with tapes or narrow bandages.[272]

Joints also has an account of humps and curvature of the spine. Most humps are incurable, especially when they are formed above the attachment of the diaphragm. But some of the low humps are said to be cured when varicosities form in the legs, particularly at the back of the knee or on the groin. This statement, whether true or not, would have been prompted by the theory of *apostasis*, or the draining of humours from one part to another. This becomes even more likely when we are told that prolonged dysentery can resolve a hump. When humps occur in children the legs and arms later grow to full size, but growth will be defective on the spine. When the hump is above the diaphragm the ribs enlarge themselves forwards, only to make a pointed chest of small capacity. The neck then has to be held concave at the great vertebra so that the head may not be thrown forward.

As a rule, hunchbacked people also have hard and unripened tubercles in the lungs, which are indeed the origin of the curvature and contraction. The same condition below the diaphragm may be complicated with ailments in the kidneys and bladder, and with purulent abscessions in the lumbar region and about the groin. Tubercles may also produce lateral curvature. The connection between tuberculosis and humps is correctly observed, perhaps for the first time in history, though the action of the tubercles is conceived to be a distorting pressure, and not, as it is known to be in our own time, a wasting of the vertebrae making the spine incapable of maintaining its normal shape against the weight of the body.

The surgeon's task was to restore the spine to its proper shape if he could, but this was usually impossible because of the tubercular wasting. One method of attempting this is strongly condemned in *Joints*, that of succussion on the ladder. The patient was bound as comfortably as possible to a ladder, feet downwards if the deformity was high on the back, head downwards if it was lower. The ladder was then raised to a vertical position against a tower or house gable, so that assistants standing on this height could lift it and let it down smoothly, neatly and vertically to strike hard ground in repeated shocks. This shaking and the pendant weight of the patient's body were expected to drag the spine out straight. There was in fact little hope of this even where the curvature was due to the shock of a fall and not to wasting of the vertebrae. In *Joints* this method is called a form of advertisement to make the vulgar herd gape and applaud. The author's own favourite apparatus is one of leverage: to make the patient lie prone by a wall on a board covered with cloaks, to pass across his hump a plank which engages at one end in a groove in the wall, and then to press down on the other end. He also recommends pressure with hand and heel.

There is a careful description of the anatomy of the spine and of the difference between curved and angular deformations, the latter being much more dangerous because of the pressure they exert on the spinal cord. There is also a description of the attachment of the ribs to the vertebrae, and of the effects of heavy blows or shocks on the ribs, bruising being considered as much as fracture of the bones.[273]

The femur presented a more serious problem. The writer

remarks that it can be dislocated from the hip in four ways, most frequently upwards, after that outwards and much less frequently backwards or forwards. When the bone is displaced inwards the leg appears longer when laid beside the other because the head of the bone is brought down and round against the ischium and supported against the lower rim of its own socket. The buttock then looks hollow on the outer side because the head of the femur is turned inwards. The lower end of the femur is forced to turn outwards at the knee, and below it the leg and foot likewise. These are the outward signs, together with an abnormal prominence at the groin caused by the head of the femur. The patient walks by bringing his dislocated leg round, as an ox does both its forelegs, and thus throws most of the weight on the sound leg, which will have its foot turned in. He requires a crutch on the side of the sound leg because the weight of the body is now inclined to that side, and is obliged to stoop because he needs to press the thigh of the dislocated leg with his hand.

Thus the body of itself finds the easiest posture. When a dislocated hip remains unreduced in a patient who has not finished growing, the thigh is maimed and the leg and foot also; the bones do not grow to normal length and the whole leg lacks flesh and muscle because it lacks proper exercise. The greatest damage is done when this joint is dislocated *in utero*, and the next greatest to those who are very young. These usually have not the energy to keep the body up in moving, but crawl about on the sound leg, supporting themselves with the hand on that side.

In outwards dislocation the leg is found to be shorter when set beside the other, for the head of the femur presses only on flesh, while the thigh on the inside appears hollow and less fleshy and the buttock is higher. The bone turns outwards at the knee, and so do the leg and foot. In walking the patient cannot reach the ground with his heel, but goes on the ball of his foot. If this lesion is neglected in the very young the whole leg becomes useless and atrophied. When the hip-joints of both legs are dislocated outwards, both legs are exercised alike, the gait is even and swaying and the haunches very prominent, while the growth of the body is defective.

In backwards dislocation of one leg the patient cannot extend his leg at the joint, though he can flex it. When walking he has to flex his body strongly at the groin because the leg is much shorter. But with practice he can walk without a crutch if he grasps and presses his thigh as required, for the sole of the foot keeps its original straight line and does not turn outwards.

In reducing inwards dislocation of the femur, the patient should be suspended by his feet from a cross-beam with a band which is strong but soft and also wide, the feet being four fingers apart or less, and should be bound round above the knee-caps with a broad soft band, the injured leg being extended two fingers' breadth further than the other. His head should be two cubits from the ground and his arms should be extended along his sides and bound with something soft. When all these preparations have been made and the patient is suspended, let a strong and skilful assistant bring down his arm between the patient's thighs to come to rest between the perineum and the head of the dislocated bone. Then, grasping the inserted hand with the other and standing erect beside the patient, let him suddenly suspend himself from him in this position and balance himself in the air as evenly as possible, while he levers out the head of the bone until it slips back into its natural place. The combined weight of the patient and the assistant will provide the necessary extension. The assistant must be very strong, and bandaging after the event perfect.[274]

As in *Fractures*, extension by apparatus, the celebrated Hippocratic bench with its various fittings, is also recommended: straps, cords and windlasses for extension, the perineal post for holding the patient against stretching of the leg, wooden levers set in any one of various grooves, and cross-bars and props. Thus a wooden lever will force a femur dislocated outwards back in. Backward dislocation should be treated by making the patient lie prone and applying extension and also downward leverage with the plank as with hunchbacks, but here on the buttock a little below the hip. Forward dislocation is most easily reduced by having the patient on his back while a strong assistant presses on his groin. Inward dislocation, again, is sometimes set right by inflating a wine skin between the closely fastened thighs of the patient. The wine skin must have been inflated with bellows, but some sort of valve would have been needed to hold in the air. There was also the use of weights, such as a basket of stones, or a jar filled with water, to produce downward extension.

One curious assertion was disputed by later surgeons and commentators. When the bone of the leg is dislocated at the knee and projects outwards or inwards, when the thigh bone is dislocated at the knee and appears through a wound, or when the elbow is dislocated in this way, these dislocations must not be reduced at once or the patient will promptly die.[275] These injuries were surely also compound fractures, as we should call them, and are recognized in modern medicine. Later writers remarked on the timidity of Hippocrates in his treatment of them.[276]

There is special mention of congenital club foot, which is said to be curable if the deviation is not great and the child very young. There are various kinds of club foot, but most cases are not complete dislocations, since they result from the foot's being kept constantly in a contracted position. In treatment the bone of the leg must be pushed inwards at the ankle, and that of the heel pressed outwards as it comes into line with the leg. The foot must be bent outwards at the same time and all the toes rotated. (At this point most manuscripts have 'bent inwards', which is the opposite of the required action, and editors have followed them. But a few manuscripts have what must be the correct reading.) The foot must be enclosed in sewn-on bandages, to maintain the required position, and a sole of leather or lead must be fastened outside the bandages.[277]

Joints also touches on the very important subject of amputation, a proceeding which must always have been in surgeons' minds if a fracture was bad enough, though it is logically out of place here. It is not treated elsewhere in our Corpus, but this may be an accident of preservation. Complete amputation of toes or fingers at the joints is said to be without danger unless the patient collapsed at the time of the injury. It is even without danger at the joints of the foot, the hand, the leg at the ankle, or the forearm at the wrist unless the patient faints away at once or falls into a continuous fever on the fourth day.

The next topic is gangrene in wounds and fractures, whether of flesh or of bone. The risk of it as well as the actual occurrence must have been a frequent reason for amputation. The complete treatise may have contained more on this subject. The writer mentions with unconcern cases where parts of the thigh or arm come away of themselves in this condition, and notes how lines of demarcation naturally arise between live and dying parts. He would rather not amputate at a place where the limb is fully alive and sentient, because there is a risk of the patient's collapsing from pain and then suddenly dying.[278] We should expect at this point some reference to control of bleeding, beyond instruction that the limb must not be left pendant. Ligation of arteries might have been beyond the techniques of the age, and the requirement for it would not have been so obvious when the nature of arteries was not understood; but some sort of tourniquet would be a natural thing to use. Here again if more had been preserved we might have found this matter treated. The modern preference for amputating at a point proximal to the gangrene and often far from it is based on our knowledge of infection and of the circulation of the blood, which is often deficient in a gangrenous limb. The pain said in *Joints* to be so dangerous is now prevented at the time of operation by anaesthetics, but there is still persisting surgical shock to be considered.

Fractures and *Joints* also contain directions for the diet and regimen of patients under treatment. An epitome of *Joints*, and of some features lost in our version of the full text, is given in *Leverage* (*Μοχλικόν*). Another surgical book in the Corpus is *Head Wounds*, which is also a most competent and practical account. The occasion of its writing was surely the experience of its author in warfare, where these injuries, rare in ordinary life, must have been extremely common whenever helmets of metal were not worn.

The most vulnerable part of the skull is the bregma, where the brain has its greatest bulk and is most sensitive, and where the bone is most likely to be fractured, contused or dented. Sharp, light weapons may make *hedrai* in the skull, that is, dents which have no fissure and no widespread contusion of the bone, but these do not of themselves cause death, even if it occurs later. But if, when the bone is denuded, a suture is revealed, then wherever the wound may be the bone offers very little resistance to injury or a weapon, and is weakest of all if the weapon actually strikes a suture.[279]

There are several modes of injury to the skull, and in the lesion there can be several forms of fracture. First, wounding of the bone may cause fracture and, generally, also contusion at the fracture and around it. Fractures can be of various shapes, depths and sizes, sometimes being too small to be noticed in time to save the patient's life. Secondly, the bone may be simply contused and keep its place, and the contusion may have varying depth, length and breadth. Thirdly, the bone may be contused and depressed inwards with fractures, the depressed part being broken away from the rest. Fourthly, a weapon may make a *hedra*, with the bone keeping its natural position and the weapon sticking into it so as to leave a mark later; there may also be fracture with contusion. Fifthly, there may be a *hedra* with contusion alone. The skull may sometimes be wounded in a different part of the head from that which has the lesion and the denuded bone, but in this case nothing can be done to help, for it cannot be discovered where this other wound is.[280]

The contusion and fissure-fracture, invisible or manifest, are cases for trepanning, and so is the *hedra* combined with these or with contusion alone. But depressed fractures with comminution require trepanning much less, and simple *hedrai* without these complications need it less still. To investigate these injuries, interrogation of the patient on all the circumstances as well as on his present feelings is no less necessary than physical examination. Probing will prove that a *hedra*, a depressed fracture or comminution exists. The most damaging wounds are deliberate, are given by a stronger man to a weaker, and result from blows meeting the skull at a right angle. Heavy hard weapons do more damage than light pointed weapons because the contusion they produce is worse than clefts or simple fractures. The pulp that they make of the scalp and outer bone will be much more purulent and will lead to more sloughing away of dead and discoloured bone. But any damage will be particularly harmful if its area covers a suture, where the bone is weaker and more porous and hence more likely to gape. A suture should never be trepanned.[281]

In treatment, plugging, plastering and bandaging are not

recommended unless incision is also needed. Incision of the scalp is mainly required for inspection purposes, incision of the bone for assisting a suitable remedy to penetrate when there is undermining of the edge of the wound. The author knows well the difference of texture between the innermost and outermost layers of bone and the marrowy layer between them. In operating, the scalp must be carefully detached from the skull where it adheres to the bone or to membranes; these membranes are thought to be the connection at the sutures between the pericranium and the *dura mater*. The whole wound must then be plugged with lint, with a plaster upon it of dough and fine barley kneaded with vinegar. If the extent and shape of the injury are still not clear the bone should be scraped up and down and crosswise with a raspatory to get a view of latent fractures. If the injury is severe and still imperfectly known a black drug should be dropped on the cleared bone, which on cleaning will appear white where it is undamaged, but will have its cracks marked in black. The wound should be made to suppurate as quickly as possible, and should then become rather dry. The membrane of the brain, when that is exposed, should also be kept as dry as possible. Any dead bone will soon flake off.[282]

In trepanning the bone should not be removed down to the membrane at once, as the latter may become macerated. Nor must the membrane ever be wounded. The trepanning instrument that the writer has in mind was a conical piece of metal with a circular serrated edge at the bottom, making it into a form of saw which cut a circular groove, and a centre pin to keep it in place as it was worked. It had a cylindrical handle several inches long which was either operated by rolling it rapidly between the palms, or according to some authorities spun by a cord and bow moved crosswise. The saw, as the author calls the trepan, had frequently to be taken out and plunged into cold water to cool because of the frictional heat. There is also mention of a perforating trepan (*τρύπανος*) which would be a simpler form of drill, used to make a ring of holes between which the bone was prised out.[283]

Trepanning or any other form of incision of the bone is not to be carried out in certain parts of the skull such as the temple, or the part above it which is traversed by the temporal blood vessel. If this is done spasms seize the patient, affecting the right side of his body if the incision is on the left side, and *vice versa.* In fatal cases, where trepanning has not been done and there is necrosis of the bone in lesions on the side of the head, there is likewise spasm on the contrary side of the body.[284] This contralateral effect was well known, though the neurological reason for it, the crossing of nerve fibres at the base of the brain, was not.

On a different level, the little book *In the Surgery* (*Κατ' ἰητρεῖον*) gives practical hints to beginners, which shows us how the surgery and its staff would appear to the patient when he came for treatment. The composition is disjointed and incomplete, and the manner and sense here and there obscure. The content on the technical side adds little to that of *Fractures* and *Joints*, and the book is regarded as a late epitome.[285]

The examining surgeon must look for differences from the normal which can be recognized by the senses. He must know how many instruments there are and how to use them, and must pay much attention to lighting; he must be placed conveniently to himself, to the part needing operation, and to the light. Both ordinary and artificial light may be used either directly or obliquely, though oblique light is rarely used. With direct light, turn the part for operation toward the brightest light, unless it is one which decency requires be not exposed. The part faces the light and the surgeon faces the part but not so as to overshadow it; thus also the part will not be exposed to view.[286] The concern for decency seems incompatible with efficient surgery, unless it is meant that others about the room, or even relatives, friends or other onlookers, should not see what is unsuitable.

The surgeon when he is seated should have his feet vertically under his knees and fairly close together, the knees a little higher than the groin and leaving room for the elbows, but still supporting them. Dress should be well drawn together without creases. The elbows should not need to pass in front of the knees or behind the ribs, nor the hands above the breast or lower, but when the chest is on the knees the forearms should be kept at right angles to the upper arms. Moving the body to right or left should be done with a suitable twist without moving the hips. The reader has the impression that Greek surgeons operated in some kind of sitting or crouching position much more often than modern ones. If he operates standing, the surgeon should make the examination with both feet fairly level, but in operating should rest the weight on one foot not on the same side as the hand that is in use. The other foot should be as high as his groin. Evidently this foot is on some high support.[287] The patient must help the surgeon by standing, sitting or lying so as to maintain most easily the proper posture without slipping, collapse, displacement or pendency. These instructions suggest that any kind of operating table was rarer then than now.

The surgeon must keep his nails neither projecting beyond the finger tips nor short of them, and practise using the finger ends with forefinger opposed to thumb, both with that hand in pronation and with both hands opposed. The hands must have well-formed fingers with wide intervals and the thumb should be easily opposable to the forefinger. All operations must be practised with each hand and both together to attain ability, grace, speed, painlessness, elegance and readiness. Since surgery is handwork (χειρουργίη) *par excellence*, the requirement for naturally well-formed and well-trained hands is obvious, as it still is for surgeons in our own time, or for musicians. The passage seems to imply deliberate exercising and care of the hands in the surgeon's spare time. Instruments must be kept conveniently near the operator's hand but not in his way, and should be handed to him by an assistant who has them ready beforehand. Those who attend on the patient should present the part for operation as needed and hold the rest of his body steady, while themselves remaining silent and obedient. Operations must be speedy, painless, resourceful and neat in their result. Bandages must be smooth and well distributed and should not disguise differences between the shape of different parts. Their varieties are simple: that is, circular, adze-shaped, rhomboid or half-rhomboid, as may suit the part and its affection.

Bandages must be firm, either by tension or by the number of them; they may sometimes be part of the cure in themselves. The pressure should be such that they neither fall away nor are very tight, but fit without forcible compression. The ends for tying must not be over the wound, but where the knot is to be. The knot must be where there is neither friction nor motion, and knots and sutures must be soft and not large.[288]

Every bandage slips towards the pendant and conical parts such as the top of the head and the bottom of the leg. Where the parts are on the right side bandages must run toward the left and *vice versa*. Holdfasts must be made on the smoothest part and must not be oblique, so that the outermost turn may hold down the most mobile one. Threaded sutures in loops to be tied at the ends or continuous sutures should be used where good fixation or support are hard to obtain.[289] In their full extent these instructions are difficult for a layman to follow, but one observation which will occur to anyone is that much trouble could have been saved in some cases if the Hippocratics had had adhesive plaster.

The functions of under-bandages are to bring together what is separated, such as the edges of a wound, to separate what is adherent, or to adjust what is distorted. Linen should be used for them; they should be thin, soft, clean and broad, and soaked in a liquid to suit each case. The liquid was no doubt intended to have healing properties like our antiseptic dressings. This was particularly needed for abscesses which continued to discharge. Instructions for the amount of bandaging are much as in other surgical books, and the same is true of splints. Instructions are also given for the use of water of suitable temperature, to be tested by pouring it over the surgeon's own hand; also for permanent positions of limbs, presentation and extension, and for massage (ἀνάτριψις). The lay reader may feel that the attention devoted to bandaging is excessive, but in various passages of the Corpus learners have to be dissuaded from treating bandages as exhibitions of skill or virtuosity in themselves.

GYNAECOLOGY AND OBSTETRICS

It seems better to treat gynaecology and obstetrics apart from general therapy and surgery, as modern medicine does. Our sources for gynaecology in the Corpus are among the most voluminous of all: *The Nature of Woman*, *Diseases of Women* in two books, with a third on *Sterile Women* (Περὶ ἀφόρων), *Super-*

foetation and *Excision of the Foetus* (*Περὶ ἐγκατατομῆς ἐμβρύου*). They are good examples of Cnidian writing.

First a word of warning may be noted from *Diseases of Women* I. All illnesses and afflictions fall for preference on women who have not had children, but sometimes they come upon those who have had them. They are serious, acute and severe, and difficult to understand because they are peculiar to women. Sometimes women do not know themselves what is wrong with them until they have experienced menstrual troubles and have reached a greater age. Thus among those who do not know the cause of their sufferings, illnesses often become incurable before the physician has been told by the patient how her illness originated. They are ashamed to speak even when they know, and from inexperience and ignorance regard it as a disgrace. Physicians on their side sometimes fail to learn accurately the exciting cause of the illness, and treat women as if they had some masculine disease. Many women have died of these illnesses for that reason. The patient must be interrogated very carefully about the cause, for women's diseases are very different from men's.[290] This passage may be called a demand for gynaecology as a special branch of medicine. In fact the gynaecological books of the Corpus go far to meet this requirement.

When we come to read them, these books show that almost every one of the common disorders now mentioned in handbooks of gynaecology were familiar to their authors. The books are full of repetitive detail and rather lacking in aetiology; they offer very little in the way of comprehensive theory, which would have had great interest for the history of science, however mistaken it might appear to us. But there are certain bizarre features which deserve special mention. For the most part the books are lists of practical descriptions and hints such as might occur in any folk medicine. But only a medical man could see the significance of many details.

To take first the common disorders. Menstruation, insufficient, excessive or irregularly timed, is mentioned explicitly in twenty-eight passages of *The Nature of Woman*, *Diseases of Women* and *Sterile Women*, much more often than any other discharge.[291] Lochial discharge after childbirth, when it is delayed or otherwise abnormal, is mentioned in eleven passages.[292] The humoral pathology is sometimes invoked to explain these irregularities, and excess of bile or phlegm in other discharges is diagnosed. The morbid discharges of leucorrhoea and metrorrhagia are described, the former in eight passages, the latter in thirteen.[293] These would constitute a large part of the material for gynaecology in any age. Conditions which would now be called metritis and vaginal inflammation are moderately common, the former being described six times.[294] The frequent mention of ulcers in various parts of the reproductive tract, fourteen references being found, is a little surprising until it is remembered how often these occurred in many parts of the body, and in both sexes, according to the Greek medical writers.[295] The reason may have been deficiencies in diet which weakened resistance to lesions or infections. Cancer, which figures prominently in modern gynaecology, is named only twice.[296] Another surprise is the prominence of dropsy in the womb, as it is called here; but this also figures in modern gynaecology.

Herbs, oil, vinegar, wine and fat from geese or cattle appear in the remedial preparations. The fats were no doubt less valuable in themselves than as a base for carrying the other ingredients.

Another condition which is often reported is hardening of the cervix, which usually closes the womb, allowing nothing to pass either way and preventing both menstruation and conception. This condition was painful and often accompanied by fever. It was treated by washing out with hot water, by fomentations and emollient pessaries of herbs and minerals wrapped in wool.[297] Carneous mole is also mentioned.[298] These disorders were attributed to faulty menstruation as the initial cause, though this was admitted to follow them even more than it preceded them.

So far the forms of illness or disorder mentioned are familiar in gynaecology, as textbooks confirm. But the many references to displacement or distortion of the womb and accompanying pains would be only partly comprehensible to a modern gynaecologist relying on anatomy and clinical evidence.[299] The oddest features are not even attributable to the feelings and statements of patients and to their ignorance of referred pain; they belong to medical theory of the time, by which the womb was regarded as a self-moving organ that could change its position to various parts of the abdomen and even further afield.

It is sometimes difficult to see how these movements were imagined; yet some of the displacements are familiar or at least conceivable. The womb is said to be displaced backwards against the viscera, to the left or to the right, obliquely, or towards the bladder.[300] Prolapse is several times mentioned.[301] Displacement to the hypochondria below the breastbone, causing vomiting and a feeling of suffocation, is alleged several times; this might be natural in some stages of pregnancy, but there is no mention of pregnancy in these passages.[302] More unlikely are displacements towards the liver or the heart.[303] But displacements said to be towards the head or the feet are odd indeed; they were believed to cause in the first case pain in the nostrils and under the eye and in the second pain in the thighs and spasms under the great toes.[304] These forms of action at a distance were nevertheless held to yield to treatment of the womb by vapour baths or fumigations, as well as of the extremities concerned.[305] In fact such peregrinations or excursions of the womb were regarded as hysteria in the original sense of affections of the womb (*ὑστέρα*), and therefore peculiar to women. This notion had a long history later in the development of neurology and psychology, and among laymen there is still some resistance to admitting that men can be hysterical.

Much of the pain and discomfort of the serious female illnesses must have been beyond the understanding of these writers because of their ignorance of the upper end of the reproductive tract: of the ovaries and their diseases, of the Fallopian tubes and their inflammation, and of such misfortunes as tubal pregnancy. Some of these troubles can issue in a general peritonitis in which abdominal pain is even more widely felt. The affections of these remoter parts, inaccessible before modern techniques of operation, may have contributed to some of the notions of displacement. Affections of the kidneys in pregnancy were recognized, but the sudden suffocations which are sometimes mentioned, and which now suggest eclampsia, were not traced to them.[306]

Some forms of gynaecological treatment have been briefly mentioned. Fumigation consisted of causing the patient to sit over a tube through which smoke rose from burning substances. Vapour baths for this purpose were also used, consisting of vessels of boiling water in which were shredded plants of medical efficacy and strong aroma.[307] Sometimes it was believed that the aroma could be detected by sniffing at the patient's head, as if the vapour could penetrate from the vagina through the entire body and head. Displacements of the womb from its normal position were usually corrected by the hand of the physician or midwife. An extreme example was succussion on the ladder, accompanied by manipulation, for reducing prolapse.[308] Dilatation was also practised, as now, for various conditions. It should be added that the pessaries mentioned were not mechanical contrivances for holding the uterus in a desired position, but remedies wrapped in wool or linen.

The gynaecological books mention more drugs than any others. One of these is *melanthion*, mentioned in *Diseases of Women* as an emmenagogue and in *Sterile Women* as a purifying pessary to help conception. If this was in fact ergot, as has been suggested, it would have another effect, that of stimulating contractions of the uterine muscles. Ergot is a fungal parasite of dark appearance found on various grasses, particularly rye. The Hippocratic author adds that *melanthion* was obtained from wheat, which is also likely enough if it was ergot.[309] Other plants mentioned – fennel, caraway, anise, myrrh, saffron, elderberry, mint, parsley, sage, camomile, cinnamon, cassia, coriander, cardamom, juniper and rue – are known as emmenagogues or diuretics.[310] Recommended as balsams are pine resin, incense, myrrh, styrax, terebinth resin, opobalsamum, sagapenum, mastic and galbanum.[311] Against hardening of the cervix, linseed and mallow are advised; against metrorrhagia and leucorrhoea, astringents such as oak bark, gallnut, pomegranate rind and acacia bark.[312] Puerperal ulcers were treated with the same oxides, sulphates and carbonates of copper as other ulcers; also with *magnetis lithos*, a silvery mineral which was perhaps a kind of talc, white lead, red lead, ruddle, alum and soda.[313]

There is very little reference to means of preventing pregnancy, as would be natural in a society where unwanted infants could be exposed. In *The Nature of Woman*, a woman desiring not to conceive is advised to soak a piece of *misy* (copper sulphate) as large as a bean in water, and to drink the liquid. She will then escape conceiving for a year.[314]

On the clearly related subject of obstetrics no separate book exists in the Corpus. This may be an accident, though this service in simpler societies than ours would in any case be in the hands of midwives, *sages-femmes* whose experience would be greater than any physician's. None the less the gynaecological books do contain a number of professional observations.

Diseases of Women mentions various maladies suffered by pregnant women. In one, menstruation continues even during pregnancy because the womb is not perfectly closed and loses blood. Treatment restores the woman's health and the growth of the foetus: otherwise she is ill and weak and any accident may bring on labour.[315] Unsuitable food, sharp or bitter, may even kill the foetus, or shock may bring it to birth premature and very weak.[316] Sudden shrinking of the breasts or belly in the seventh or eighth month of pregnancy is a sign that the foetus is dead or very weak.[317] In birth, presentation that is oblique or by the feet is worst. The births of dead children, of apoplectic ones or of twins are very difficult.[318]

Some further hints are as follows. To bring out the after-birth, useful remedies are wormwood, dittany, white violet flowers and silphium, all taken internally.[319] When a foetus has been dead for one or two months it is necessary to fatten the mother before it can be presented.[320] Surgical means of bringing out a dead infant by section of its body are described, and also drugs to be administered for this purpose: galbanum in oil of cedar wrapped in linen to be applied to the orifice, and many more such as hellebore and cantharidies, all stimulants and irritants.[321] *Superfoetation* describes awkward presentations: arms and legs appearing first must be pushed back again; the head appearing while the rest remains fixed shows a dangerous situation, for which, oddly enough, fumigation is proposed as treatment.[322] There are more such details, but in no book is there an account of a normal birth and of procedure such as a midwife would follow.[323] But neither are there any accounts of monsters. It is evident that Hippocratic medicine faced every obstetrical emergency, whether successfully or not. In these books there is no refusal to treat a patient, as in some that deal with other branches.

MEDICAL ETHICS, ETIQUETTE AND MANNER WITH PATIENTS

After so much of a technical nature, this chapter may conclude with the purely human aspect of medicine as shown in the Corpus. Some writings under this head are well known to literary scholars, particularly the celebrated Oath, which will be considered first.[324]

The Hippocratic Oath in some form has been known to the medical profession in countries of European culture, and even among Jews and Arabs, since Greek times, but the forms in which it has been administered have often been different from the original Greek one, particularly in modern times, when indeed any such general undertaking in explicit words has been growing rarer. The Greek text contains various elements in its short extent: directions on medical ethics, referring to the patient's family as well as to the patient himself; an undertaking not to practise surgery; a covenant to respect and if necessary to teach other members of the profession; and finally an element which seems not only moral but religious. These will be considered in that order, which is not the order of the text.

The Oath was probably taken at the end of his training by a young man who may be compared to a qualified physician. He swears to apply dietetic measures for the benefit of the sick according to his ability and judgment, and to keep them from harm and injustice. The importance of diet has been amply illustrated in the other books; the harm and injustice may refer to what the patient would inflict on himself through unhealthy living and feeding. The vow not to give a deadly drug to anyone if asked for it, and not to give a woman an abortive remedy, seems to be a special addition to ordinary medicine, for in Greek life and medical practice neither suicide nor abortion were forbidden. The explanation may be in the next sentence, where the beginner promises to guard his life and his art in purity and holiness. These words sound odd in a purely medical context. To promise not to commit any intentional injustice in any house visited, and to abstain from sexual relations with both female and male persons, free or slaves, will be acknowledged to be normal ethics in the profession. Indulgence in these things is still the commonest meaning assumed for the phrase 'infamous conduct in a professional respect'. Some scholars have found difficulty in the undertaking not to spread abroad anything seen or heard in the course of treatment or even outside it in the life of men. In our age, when there are other confidential professions such as banking and solicitor's practice, there is little reason for misunderstanding this. The question is one of life and circumstances, not of logical subdivision. The undertaking not to use the knife, not even on sufferers from stone, but to leave this to professionals in that work is again an addition or special restriction, setting up a stricter division than usual between physicians and surgeons. It seems to apply to operative surgery. The treatment of fractures and dislocations would not be barred, but only some kinds of surgery, including abortion, which appear in the Hippocratic books. However, surgery in general is not here condemned as wrong or unworthy, but simply set aside as different.

The covenant which the young man makes binds him to hold his teacher the equal of his parents and the partner of his life, to help him with money if he needs it, to treat his sons as if they were his own brothers and to teach them medicine free of charge or covenant if they desire to learn it, to give his own sons and his teacher's sons a share in the precepts, oral instruction, and all other instruction, and to instruct in the same way pupils who have signed and sworn according to the medical rule, but not anyone else. It has sometimes been argued that this shows that medicine was definitely based on medical families which could add members by adoption, and that the model of such families was that of the Asclepiads, who had once been the only possessors of medicine; also that among families of craftsmen this practice was the rule in archaic training and education. There is not enough evidence for this, however, except among the Pythagorean brotherhood, who were like the religious orders of later times, though not celibate.

The religious language concerning purity and holiness, the

undertaking not to practise surgery, which required the drawing of blood, and also the refusal of help for suicide or abortion could be Pythagorean features also. They made the Oath especially acceptable to Christianity, Judaism and Islam, among those civilizations which maintained the Greek tradition of medicine. The Pythagorean texts from which these useful analogies come are not earlier than the fourth century, and somewhere in this period is likely to be the date of the Oath. Thus the Oath was not originally framed for all physicians, but for some who had been strongly influenced by the Pythagoreans. Though the Pythagorean brotherhood in southern Italy had been broken up by this time, its doctrines continued to be spread beyond that region by individuals. This is at least a tenable theory, which explains the peculiarities of the Oath.

Other writings on the ethical and social aspects of the medical profession are found in the Corpus as we have it. Though they appear to be later than the Hippocratic age proper and show traces of Aristotelian ethics or Hellenistic philosophy, they were gathered into the Corpus for their content in ancient times, and it is most convenient to discuss them here.

The nearest in interest to the Oath is the little tract called *Law* (*Νόμος*), which sets out the necessary elements in the education of a good physician.[325] It claims that medicine is the most illustrious of all the skills, but because of the ignorance both of its practitioners and of others who judge it casually it is now the least esteemed. The chief reason is that states have made failure subject to no penalty but that of dishonour. This does not wound false practitioners, who are like supernumeraries in tragedies as contrasted with real actors. As these are dressed as actors without being actors, so quacks are physicians by repute but not in fact. (In the lack of penalties for malpractice we notice an important difference from the professional discipline of our own time, which is maintained within the profession and approved by the state.) To acquire skill in medicine, natural ability is required and also prolonged teaching and application; these elements are like the soil, the seed and the work of cultivation in the growing of plants. Real knowledge of the art is required before we can travel from city to city and win a reputation in deeds. But things which are holy are revealed only to men who are holy and have been initiated into the mysteries of science. The last words have been held to imply an actual ritual of initiation into a craft or guild, and the tone suggests Stoic influence.

More mundane is *The Physician* (*Περὶ ἰητροῦ*), which begins with hints on manner and deportment.[326] The physician should have as good a colour and plumpness as nature intended, for most people think that a man in poor condition will not take good care of others. He should be clean in person, well-dressed and anointed with sweet-smelling unguents that arouse no suspicion. He must be silent and very regular in his life, which will enhance his reputation; he must be a gentleman in character, grave and humane, for too much forwardness and obtrusiveness is despised, even though it may be very useful. Let him be careful of the licence that he enjoys, for the same treatment is acceptable only when the same circumstances occur rarely. (This sentence is difficult; it appears to mean that unvarying treatment and behaviour can appear insensitive if repeated often.) In the expression of his face let him be gravely thoughtful but not harsh, for then he will appear to be arrogant and unkind. But a man who readily relaxes into laughter and is too merry is assumed to be vulgar, and that is particularly to be avoided. He must be fair and be seen to take the side of fairness. His relation with patients is very intimate. Patients put themselves into the hands of their physicians, and at every moment he meets women, maidens and possessions very precious indeed, towards which he must use self-control.

Directions follow for the lighting and other arrangements of the surgery: they are like those given in *In The Surgery*. Strong daylight striking directly in the patient's face is bad, for it may trouble a patient with weak eyes. Water must be clean; bandages must not be over-elaborate; operations must be done at the right speed, which will be different in different cases. The use of surgical knives and cupping glasses is described. A word is said of ligating the vessels of the forearm in bleeding; directions for treating wounds and ulcers are given. The moral, social and technical aspects of common practice are thus set out in combination for the guidance of a student apprentice. The details concerning personal appearance and manner have a Hellenistic flavour which rather recalls Theophrastus' *Characters* and New Comedy.

Decorum (Περὶ εὐσχημοσύνης) is another writing which is shown by the peculiar Greek to be of late date.[327] It also has a philosophical flavour in certain passages which confirm the impression. Medicine is called a form of wisdom (σοφίη) applied to life and directed towards decorum and good repute. Any wisdom having some scientific method is honourable if it is not tainted with a base love of gain and unseemliness, so as to become popular through impudence. Such behaviour is the delight of young men, but when they are grown up they are ashamed, and when they are old pass laws to banish quacks from their cities. The wise men that we need would show the opposite behaviour. They should dress simply, without elaboration, in a style adapted for contemplation, introspection and walking – details which suggest a self-conscious philosopher as the model for the practitioner to imitate. These medical sages are expected to be concentrated in their work, free of extravagances, sharp in encounters, ready with replies, hard against opposition, but with those of like mind sharp-witted and affable; even-tempered towards all, silent in the face of disturbance; in the face of silence ready with arguments and persistent, ready for a chance and quick to grasp it; economical and free from addiction in the use of food, patient in waiting for an opportunity. They must set out in cogent language everything that has been suggested by examination. They must be graceful in speech, gracious in disposition, strong in the reputation that comes of these qualities, making truth their goal when it has been indicated. The sense of many of these phrases is uncertain, for some of the words are hardly found elsewhere. Here again there seems to be influence from some form of technical language used in ethical theory of the Hellenistic period.

The author continues by claiming that nature is the dominant thing among all the qualities mentioned, and also that the art, like wisdom, is not a thing that can be taught. This should mean that there is no substitute for actual practice; instruction cannot do everything. If nature is defective in any learner or practitioner, skill in speaking and ready opinions not tested in action are but a sign of want of education and of art. In medicine mere opining brings particular blame. (This recalls the Stoic who knows and never opines, but again the whole passage is obscure.)

A physician who is a lover of wisdom is the equal of a god. There is no separation between wisdom and medicine. Medicine has in it all the requirements for wisdom: indifference to gain, steadfastnesss, modesty, humility, sound opinion, judgment, quietness, facing up to opponents, purity, brief and weighty speech, knowledge of things good and necessary for life, riddance of unclean things, freedom from superstition, divine pre-eminence. Those who have it know how to manage their incomes and how to treat their children. A further passage of great difficulty seems to assert that medicine is honoured by the gods, but that the gods are the real physicians, with whom physicians co-operate in all their forms of treatment. Practical advice is given next in the usual terms on palpation, instruments, drugs and other remedies, on composure, dignity and self-control at the patient's bedside, and on the authority that the physician needs. It is also recommended that a pupil shall be left in charge to carry out instructions and administer the treatment, keeping a careful watch on the patient. This is a hint of the provision for nursing beyond the powers of the family.

The last of these books to be considered is *Precepts* (Παραγγελίαι), which again is late in date and exceedingly obscure in places, and is moreover a patchwork of originally unconnected pieces.[328] Certain new points alone need mention. There should be no discussion of fees during the illness, for that will suggest that you will leave the patient if no agreement is reached, or at least neglect to propose immediate treatment. Such a worry will be harmful to the patient, particularly if the disease is acute. It is better to reproach a patient whom you have saved than to extort money from a man mortally sick. That this piece of advice should be thought necessary shows that there were many physicians who lacked even a minimum of consideration and psychological skill. The young physician is advised sometimes to give his services for nothing, and particularly to assist a stranger if he is short of money. For where there is love of man, there is also love of the art. Some patients, though they know that their condition is perilous, are contented with the goodness of the physician and make the change to recovery.

Quacks on the other hand take all credit for recovery, but if there is a relapse merely stand upon their dignity. They do not attempt treatment when they see an alarming condition, and will not call in other physicians because they wickedly hate help. In perplexity the physician should call others into consultation; on such occasions physicians must never quarrel or jeer at one another. Jealousy is a sign of weakness. The patient's hopes must be maintained and he must be told not to worry. If you wish to give a lecture to a crowded audience this is no laudable ambition, but you should at least avoid quotations from the poets, for this shows weakness in industry. Voluble and flowery language and a parade of definitions when in charge of a case are a late learner's faults. (If this is the sense, it indicates that the profession was infested with quacks attempting to learn in a hurry, and to make themselves impressive.)

These books dealing with medical ethics show that, except in the important matter of enforceable discipline for members, something like a modern profession was gradually being created, with practitioners who were expected to be more than efficient craftsmen. The growing insistence on inner attitude after the Hippocratic age was an important advance in medicine. Such standards, which have been regarded as second nature for a good physician later in civilized ages, needed an effort to conceive and to attain, and much of the credit should go to the ethical thought of the philosophical schools. It is unfortunate that we have not more ethical doctrine surviving from the Hippocratic age itself, for then the measure of this advance could be taken. But if we had this information it is probable that the change would still be found great enough. Thus from the fourth century onwards philosophy in the form of ethics had an effect on medicine no less important than the earlier influence of another of its branches, that of speculation about nature.[329]

At this point we take leave of the Hippocratic Corpus and its accretions. Not all the books have been used for the account just concluded. The material of *Aphorisms* and other such books is indeed valuable, but it is largely identical with that found in the continuous books. These collections of short sayings cannot be reduced to summaries because their contents are too varied and disconnected. Nor is the numerical lore of such a book as *Sevens* (*Περὶ ἑβδομάδων*) worth reproducing. The Corpus has been presented in its subject-matter as the basis on which later medicine rested. The Alexandrian discoveries and other alterations are hardly conceivable without it. How much of value was never included in the Corpus we cannot know for certain, but it is representative enough of the first great age of medicine.

CHAPTER V

MEDICINE BETWEEN THE HIPPOCRATICS AND THE ALEXANDRIANS

Before we pass on to the Alexandrians, the work and thought of some other figures must be noticed. These are once more named persons, but their writings, with one exception, survive mainly in fragments.

The exception is Plato. His *Timaeus* contains a long medical and physiological section on the origin and nature of the human body within the framework of his cosmology, which owes much to the Pythagoreans and something to Empedocles.[330] Like every other section of Platonic science concerning the phenomenal world that the *Timaeus* contains, this medical section is to be understood as an imperfect account, not merely because of human ignorance of fact, but because everything in this world is intrinsically approximate and imperfect compared with the rational model in the world of forms, so that the most accurate knowledge falls short of the perfect knowledge that can be had only of a perfect object of thought. Plato has something of the same attitude to the empirical world as Parmenides had before him, in his rather perfunctory account of the world of seeming as contrasted with true being. The content of this section of the *Timaeus* can in parts be used as evidence for the continuing thought of the Siceliote and Italiote physicians mentioned in Chapter 3, whom Plato met on his western visits.

Perhaps peculiar to Plato is the attempt to find physical lodging for his well-known parts of the soul, mortal or immortal. Indeed this is the reason for the interest in physiology he shows here. The mortal parts of the soul are accommodated in the body from the neck downwards. The courageous and spirited part is in the upper chest above the diaphragm, where it can listen to reason and help it to subdue the rest. The actual guardhouse where this part dwells is the heart, the junction of the vessels and the fount of the circulating blood. When reason passes the word round to every organ that something wrong is being done in the heat of passion, the heart leaps and grows hot, but is cooled by the lungs, which are soft and bloodless and absorb the excess of heat, making it easier for the heart in its excitement to serve the reason. Below the diaphragm is the seat of the appetitive soul, which is necessary for life but needs to be kept chained and remote from the seat of reason. This part of the soul is controlled through the liver, which is dense, smooth, bright and sweet, though it contains bitterness also, and answers to thoughts from the mind. Threats from the mind move the bile, and paint bilious colours on the liver's surface. The lobe of the liver is then compressed and bent so as to block the passage and gates leading from it, causing pains and nausea. A breath of mildness from the mind, on the other hand, paints on the liver appearances of the opposite kind and uses the sweetness of the liver to smooth and straighten all its parts, so that the part of the soul planted round the liver is cheerful and serene; it occupies its slumbers with divination, since it has no share in reasoning. In this account of the liver as the organ of divination Plato is using ancient ideas which contain no element of rational medicine, but are linked with the oriental practice of hepatoscopy, divination by the appearance of the liver in sacrificed animals.

On the left of the liver the spleen has the function of keeping it bright and clean, like a wiper always ready for a mirror. When impurities due to ailments gather round the liver the loose texture of the spleen, porous and bloodless, absorbs them, so that it grows large and festering until the body is cleansed, when it settles back into its original state.

The length and curvature of the entrails, which hold superfluous meat and drink, is intended to prevent food from passing through them too quickly and causing insatiate appetite which would make mankind impervious to culture and philosophy. It is strange to find Plato not seeking a purely physiological reason for the extent of the entrails in the requirements of complete digestion.

The spinal marrow is called the universal 'seed-stuff' for every mortal kind, containing the bonds which fasten the soul or principle of life to the body. By the physical theory earlier set out, it consists of primary triangles or surfaces of primary tetrahedrons of which the simple solids in matter are composed. On a larger scale this seed-stuff has been formed into the shapes of organs capable of receiving the several kinds of soul. Such is the spinal marrow, which at one end of the spine is moulded into a globular mass, the brain, contained in a framework of bone. Later the expression spermatic marrow is used of it. Once more we have something like the doctrine of Alcmaeon, that the semen comes from the brain and marrow. The belief accounts for the primary living quality of the spinal marrow as here conceived. In modern physiology all this is not semen but nervous tissue, the vehicle of sensation and motor response, as Alcmaeon in his fashion also saw. But one reason for this confusion might be the cerebro-spinal fluid. The brain in the *Timaeus* is thus naturally the seat of the rational or intellectual element of the soul. But this seat is not so very clearly emphasized as are the corresponding seats of the soul's elements. In the basic physiology of Plato there is no clear distinction between nerve tissue and semen as the essential stuff of life, for nerve tissue was not yet clearly recognized in its true nature.

The spinal marrow below the head is protected by jointed vertebrae, but for greater protection and flexibility sinews and flesh are added, for they protect particularly against heat and cold, and against shock, as in falling. No distinction appears, such as is recognized in the Hippocratic *Fleshes*, between spinal marrow and bone marrow, for a special degree of life is thought to be inherent in all bones. The rest of the body is thus regarded largely as a padded casing for the tissue that we call nerve tissue and its enclosing bone. The real nature of the protecting flesh is so little considered that the muscles and their functions are ignored. Nor is any other nervous tissue than that of the brain and spinal cord recognized here, least of all the nerves that serve the muscles, which are hard to see.

Nutrition and respiration are combined in a curious pattern. Respiration, keeping the internal fire of the body constantly in motion, enables the body's particles of fire to penetrate and cut up the food and drink in the stomach. It thus brings about the chemical process of digestion, as we call it; the action of heat was always important in ancient theories of digestion, which was conceived as a kind of cooking.

Respiration also drives the nutritive blood, which has picked up the liquid products of the belly, about the system. A current of air breathed out through the pores is replaced by an intake through the porous skin of the chest, and so too the current breathed out in ordinary expiration through the windpipe is replaced by an intake in the reverse direction by the same route. If this interpretation is correct, there are two rhythms of respiration, one by the pores, the other by the windpipe.

Disease occurs first through excess or deficiency of one of the elements, earth, air, fire and water, and through misplacement of these in the body. A second class occurs when substances such as marrow, bone, flesh and sinew, formed of the elements in various proportions, become corrupted and the process of their formation is reversed. The products of this decomposition are carried everywhere through the vessels, feuding among themselves and at war with everything in the body that keeps its orderly array and position. These inharmonious humours, bile, acid phlegm and white phlegm, engender disease whenever the blood is not replenished naturally from meat and drink. A third class of diseases arises from blockage of inspired air in the blood vessels and round the sinews and tendons, which causes convulsions, and from blockage of white phlegm and black bile resulting in inflammations. These morbid humours overcome the fibrine in the blood and eventually dissolve the marrow, the basis of life, thus causing death. There is a final paragraph on fevers: quotidians are due to excess of air, tertians to excess of water, and quartans to excess of earth. The fevers seem to be initiated by an excess of fire.

This account of physiology and pathology is introduced not

for its own sake but as a help in the care of the soul. At all points it is treated as merely probable. In other dialogues, too, Plato makes many references to medicine, but always in order to draw comparisons between the care of the body and his real interest, the care of the soul. Yet this part of the *Timaeus* is deemed worthy of summary in *Anonymus Londinensis*.[331]

Analogies to various Hippocratic books suggest themselves but cannot be pressed. It is rather to later medicine that Plato may be indebted, as appears in the fragmentary information that we have on the views of some physicians of the Western medical school. Philolaus of Croton, for instance, is reported in *Anonymus Londinensis* to have taught that our bodies are composed of heat.[332] Semen is warm, and so is the womb where it is deposited. When the newborn child inhales the external air, which is cold, it discharges it again like a debt, but our bodies continue to need inhaled air to cool their heat. He holds that disease arises through bile, blood and phlegm. The blood is rendered thick when the flesh is compressed inwards, but becomes thin when the vessels in the flesh are broken up. He also says that bile is serum of flesh, and denies that it has its station in the liver. He calls phlegm hot because its name is derived from *phlegein* 'to burn'. Thus it is by participation in phlegm that inflamed parts are inflamed. Contributory causes are excesses of heat, of nutriment, of chill. An important feature of Philolaus' theory is that the humours, which in most of the Hippocratic Corpus are normal constituents of the body which can become unbalanced, are morbid products not present in the healthy body. Certainly this is also the impression that we have from the account of them in the *Timaeus*.

Another Western physician, whom Plato met in Syracuse, was Philistion of Locri in southern Italy, whose views are likewise reported in *Anonymus Londinensis*.[333] Philistion's physics was of the Empedoclean kind, using the four forms, fire, air, water and earth as elements, that is, hot, cold, moist and dry respectively. Diseases he traced to three main kinds of cause: the elements, the condition of our bodies, and external causes. The elements cause disease when, for instance, the hot and moist are in excess, as when the hot becomes too weak in the body. The condition of the body causes disease when breathing is checked throughout its length; when the breath passes well and freely, health is the result. For breathing takes place not only in the mouth and nostrils, but all over the body. This would be the doctrine of respiration through the skin, which corresponds to some facts known to modern medicine – for complete blocking of all the pores has been found to cause death. The influence of Philistion on the *Timaeus* appears to be strong and definite, and Plato was not the only writer to be indebted to him.

Another Western physician was Timotheus of Metapontion in southern Italy.[334] He held a view of digestive residues as the cause of disease, very much in the Egyptian and Cnidian manner, but believed that the effects were particularly mediated through the head. When the head is clear, the nutriment from the whole body is added to it and the creature is healthy, but when the head is not healthy, it causes disease because of the passage of phlegm about the body. When the passages are blocked, the residue mounts to the head and finds no issue. Remaining there, it changes to salty and acrid moisture and finally forces a breach, so that it reaches other parts. The nature of the disease caused is determined by the position of the part affected; for instance when the moisture is collected in the windpipe it produces choking and short gasps – this sounds like asthma. The head may be diseased through an excess of chill or heat or through a blow. This account of disease seems to add to the doctrine of residues something like the doctrine of fluxes of phlegm which appears, for example, in *The Sacred Disease*. The Western physicians are likely to have followed Empedocles in believing that the heart and not the brain was the seat of consciousness.

A similar doctrine of morbid discharges from the head was held by an unknown physician named Aias or Abas, also mentioned in *Anonymus Londinensis*.[335]

In the same source Thrasymachus of Sardis, otherwise unknown, is quoted as making blood the source of diseases: through excess of cold or heat blood changes to phlegm, bile or pus, which bring disease.[336] Here again the humours, other than blood, which is sometimes reckoned one of them, are treated as morbid products.

So too Dexippus of Cos is reported to have thought that

diseases arise from residues of unsuitable nutriment which stir up bile and phlegm.[337] These cause disease by their quantity, position or form, and so do excesses of heat or cold or similar things. Dexippus added that bile and phlegm can meet, producing sera and sweats which then thicken into pus, resulting in noise in the ears, mucus and rheum. Other variations on surfeit and residues due to undigested food forming unhealthy fluids are found in the unknown Phasias of Tenedos and in Aegimius of Elis.[338]

A more important figure than any of these is Diocles of Carystus in Euboea, the first medical writer to use Attic, and a pupil of Aristotle.[339] He is cited by Theophrastus but not mentioned at all in *Anonymus Londinensis*, though the writer of this papyrus claims to use material descending from Aristotle and his school.[340] Like Plato in the *Timaeus* he shows the influence of Empedocles and Philistion, whose opinions he combines with Hippocratic doctrines. Material for reconstructing his theories comes from Galen and Pliny, and also from an anonymous manuscript and the *De Semine* of Vindicianus, in origin a translation from Greek.[341] The physiology of Diocles is once more based on the four elements of Empedocles, and their fundamental qualities heat, moisture, dryness and cold. Heat is of great importance in forming the humours, blood, phlegm, yellow and black bile. This heat is innate and works on the nutriment taken by the vessels from the stomach: blood is the normal result of this process, bile of an excess of heat, phlegm of a deficiency of it. Bile causes inflammation, phlegm, catarrhs. There are also the usual external causes for disease. Like Philistion, and Plato in the *Timaeus*, he makes *pneuma* an essential cause of health or sickness. Unlike the heat, it has to be drawn in from outside through the windpipe, the oesophagus, and the pores of the skin. Once within the body, *pneuma* has its seat in the heart, the governing organ, just as heat has, and is distributed from there through the body.[342] It is the active power that carries the body, and the body is passively carried by it. When the humours block the vessels through which it should pass there is disease or death.[343]

Blocking by phlegm causes an unnatural chilling and fixation of the blood; bile on the other hand makes the blood boil and then thicken. The *pneuma* in either case is hindered in its movement and produces fever as a supervening disorder. The *pneuma* is supplemented by other *pneuma* taken in with food and in breathing, which serves to cool the inner heat, and by perspiration through the pores, some invisible, some visible. Perspiration in drops he regards as an unnatural condition. From the heart, which is still the main organ of sensation and thought as in Empedocles, *pneuma* streams out to the organs of sense to cause perception. Delirium resulting from phrenitis or inflammation of the diaphragm he explains by saying that the inflammation spreads from the diaphragm to affect the heart. The heart is the source of all blood. Like some writers in the Hippocratic Corpus Diocles distinguishes between the thick *arteria* and the other vessels, called *phlebes*. The *arteria* stretches to the kidneys and bladder and carries the heart's blood and *pneuma* from all sources. Other vessels, both deep-seated and superficial, also carry both, as do those of the liver, lungs and abdomen.[344]

As in Empedocles and in the *Timaeus* respiration is a process set going by the movements of the blood, and takes place both through the mouth and nose and through the pores; as air is breathed out through the mouth and nose it comes in through the pores, and as it is exhaled through the pores it comes in through the mouth and nose.[345]

Nutriment is distributed through the body by the vessels that run outward from the stomach and in the normal state convey residues to the bowel. When the blood is excessively heated and thickened in the vessels leading out of the stomach the contents are held there undigested. Phlegm and its resulting cold also prevent digestion, and the blood curdles or turns to water. Fermentation or putrefaction of food in the stomach due to heat is digestion, which depends on a balanced mixture of foods and the *pneuma* that they contain; when this is broken up there is indigestion.[346]

Bile, when it is separated out in the liver, forces its way into the gall-bladder through vessels the blocking of which causes jaundice. The kidneys separate out urine through the ureters. Good digestion sharpens the senses. The cold of winter and the heat of summer can be mitigated in their effects by food of contrary character. But in the different seasons, and for the different sexes and ages of man, particular mixtures of qualities are suitable. This principle underlies the distinctions that he makes in prescribing diets.[347]

Diocles followed Empedocles in his embryology too. For him male and female seed both contribute to the embryo, and seed comes from the brain and spinal marrow. Hence he concludes that an excess of sexual intercourse damages the eyes and marrow. Semen is made by nourishment, as Hippocrates said in his book *Nutrition* (*Περὶ τροφῆς*). The full development of the embryo takes forty days; after the twenty-seventh of these faint traces of the head and backbone can be seen enclosed in a moist integument. Boys develop faster than girls – like Empedocles, he must have based this claim on another, that they grow on the right side, which is warmer. In Pythagorean fashion he regards cycles of seven years as important in human development after birth. He thinks the embryo viable as early as the seventh month; so that a child born in the eighth month may live, but is weak and liable to die. Infertility in women he attributes to absence or deficiency of seed, to lack of the element that should form a foetus, to lack of heat, cold, moisture or dryness, or to paralysis of the womb. In men he gives similar causes, adding abnormal direction and disproportionate size of the genitals. The infertility of female mules he ascribes to small size, narrowness, and bad positioning in the womb, of which he had dissected specimens. This piece of reasoning was taken by Galen as a sign that his imperfection in human anatomy was due to purely animal dissection. Diocles was among those who believed that the blood vessels of the womb ended in teat-like structures within it which were sucked by the embryo. Like Empedocles, he thought that menstruation in all women covered the same span of years, from the fourteenth to the sixtieth.[348]

In gynaecology Diocles held that chill in the shins and a feeling of heaviness in the back were signs of miscarriage to be expected. Broad hips, red hair and a mannish aspect were for him infallible signs of fertility, which could also be confirmed by fumigation. The smoke or vapour being perceptible in the mouth or head would indicate that passages of the body were not obstructed. For difficult birth the following were causes: a defective or dead foetus, a transverse position, hardening and closing of the mouth of the womb, a moist and warm constitution, and first pregnancy.[349]

Like the Hippocratics Diocles attended to prognosis; Galen remarks on his study of urine, and on his belief in critical days, particularly the seventh and those following at intervals of seven. Morbid matter passed through three stages: an unconcocted raw state, concoction, and crisis or riddance.[350]

He wrote on diet, in particular a work of instruction in several books, *Directions on Health for Plistarchus* (Ὑγιεινὰ πρὸς Πλείσταρχον), in which he corrected the Hippocratic *Regimen* in several points. Thus in the first book he remarks that foods should not be discussed in terms of the causes of their distinctive properties, such as smell and flavour, but in terms of their observed effects on nutrition and digestion, on the belly and on urine and the humours – that is to say, in modern terms, that similar sensible properties in them, however caused, do not imply similar chemical action. Nor does he accept the dietetic methods of Herodicus, already condemned in *Epidemics* and in Plato. He is not in favour of the usual vomiting after meals, because nature already provides adequate evacuation for excesses of food and drink. But he does not deny the usefulness of emetics in treatment for special purposes, and even gives some prescriptions. He recommends sexual intercourse for cold, moist and atrabilious constitutions, but only within limits, particularly in youth and old age, for excess will damage the bladder, kidneys, lungs, eyes and backbone. Exercise and nourishment should be kept in balance; the details are much as in the Hippcratic books of regimen.[351]

In Diocles' pathology, abnormalities in *pneuma* and in the humours were main considerations. He explained fevers by an increase in heat due to wounds, inflammations, buboes and stoppage of *pneuma*. He prescribed venesection in the arm and under the tongue, but only for the strong and full-blooded. Lethargy he traced to chilling of the *pneuma* in heart and brain caused by curdling of the blood, and prescribed no baths but acid drinks, massage and sternutatories. Epilepsy he explained by phlegm which blocked the flow of *pneuma*; this was created by an excess of wine and meat in the diet. He prescribed venesection after the first onset, and then change of diet; also physical exercise, diuretics, aperient pills, emetics, vinegar and sternutatories before sleep.[352] Diocles' explanations and recommended treatments of phrenitis, apoplexy, pleurisy, pneumonia, stoppage of the bowels, dropsy and other diseases mentioned in Hippocratic pathology include nothing new.

In the history of pharmacology he has a place because of his book *Rhizotomika* (Ῥιζοτομικά), in which he was the first to make a list of plants with their effects on the human body. This is the beginning of a tradition which lasts until Dioscorides; it was used by Theophrastus for his *History of Plants*. Diocles appears also to have been the first systematic writer on anatomy; his work may have been used by Aristotle. His works were: *On Fire and Air* (*Περὶ πυρὸς καὶ ἀέρος*), *Anatomy* (*Ἀνατομή*), *Hints on Health for Plistarchus*, *On Digestion* (*Περὶ πέψεως*), *On Fevers* (*Περὶ πυρετῶν*), *On Women's Diseases* (*Περὶ γυναικείων*), *On Bandages* (*Περὶ ἐπιδέσμων*), *On the Equipment of a Surgery* (*Περὶ τῶν κατ' ἰητρεῖον*), *Prognostic* (*Προγνωστικόν*), *On Treatment* (*Περὶ θεραπειῶν*), *Sickness, Causes and Treatment* (*Πάθος αἰτία θεραπεία*), *Rhizotomica*, *On Vegetables* (*Περὶ λαχάνων*), *On Lethal Drugs* (*Περὶ θανασίμων φαρμάκων*), *Archidamus* (*Ἀρχίδαμος*), a discussion of his father's views on oil for massage and anointing.[353]

These writings of Diocles are represented only by fragments. The only piece of greater length has more than a medical interest. It is written in the form of a letter entitled *Diocles to King Antigonus* (*Διοκλῆς ἐπιστολὴ προφυλακτική*).[354] (Now that Diocles is dated as a younger contemporary of Aristotle, there is no reason to regard it as a forgery, as was once done. The king addressed would be the first Macedonian king of that name to claim rule over Greece, namely Antigonus the One-eyed, who lived from 382 to 301 BC.) The letter promises to tell the king, as the most cultured of all the kings and the longest acquainted with philosophy, including medicine, whence diseases arise, what are the warning signs, and how measures can be taken to help.

First, four regions of the body are defined: head, thorax, intestines and bladder. (These must be the parts that are specially vulnerable to disease, while 'body' is used to mean the trunk only.) Premonitory signs in the head are giddiness, headache and heaviness in the brows, singing in the ears, pricking in the temples; also tears in the eyes on rising, dullness of sight, failure of the sense of smell and swelling of the gums. For these a boiled concoction of hyssop and organy is recommended, to be swallowed on an empty stomach and used also as a mouth-wash and a gargle to reduce inflammation. Mustard with warm honeyed water is also good to swallow and gargle to reduce the streaming phlegm, after the head has been covered and warmed. The signs described suggest to us perhaps a heavy cold or influenza. But neglect of them will result in ophthalmia, glaucoma, bursting discharge from the ears, scrofulous swellings of the neck, mortification of the brain, heavy catarrh, an acute soreness of the throat at night, swollen uvula, loss of hair, ulceration of the head and toothache.

Signs of coming trouble in the thorax are: sweat over the whole body and the thorax, thickness of the tongue, spitting of salty, bitter or bilious matter, unaccountable pains under the ribs and shoulder-blades, continual yawning, sleeplessness, breathlessness, thirst after sleep, mental gloom, pulsation in the chest and arms, trembling of the hands and dry coughs. Useful remedies against these are vomiting after dinner without surfeit or drugs, also vomiting on a low diet, or *syrmaismos*, after swallowing radishes, cardamom, rocket, mustard, purslane and some warm water. Neglect of these signs will result in pleurisy, pneumonia, melancholia, acute fever, phrenitis, lethargy and burning fever with hiccups.

For trouble in the intestines the warning signs are as follows. The gut is twisted about itself and disturbed; food and drink taste bitter; there is heaviness in the knees; bending at the loins is impossible; there are causeless pains all over the body, numbness in the legs, light fever. Against these the intestines should be made soft by diet without drugging. Safe foods are beetroot boiled in honeyed water, boiled garlic, mallow, monk's rhubarb, mercury and honey cakes, all of which loosen the bowels; for exacerbation of any of these signs mix safflower with all the boiled dishes. Smooth cabbage boiled in plenty of water is also helpful; the juice of this should be drunk with honey and salt, or the water from boiled chickpea or bitter vetch, on an empty stomach. Those who neglect these signs are threatened with diarrhoea, dysentery, lientery, ileus, sciatica, tertian fever, gout, apoplexy, piles and arthritis.

For serious trouble developing in the bladder the signs are these: a feeling of fullness after very little food, gaseous distension, belching, bad colour all over the body, heavy sleep, white and scanty urine, swellings round the genitals. They must be countered with diuretic spices – roots of fennel and parsley soaked in sweet white wine, of which two cupfuls should be drunk with water early each day, daucus, myrrh or calamint. Water in which vetches have been boiled should be taken in the same way with wine. Neglect of these signs is followed by dropsy, enlarged spleen, pain about the liver, bladder-stone, nephritis, stranguria and a burning sensation in the gut. Use gentle treatment with infants and more drastic with older people.

Seasonal diet is also prescribed on the principle *contraria contrariis*. From the winter solstice until the spring equinox the prevailing catarrh must be counteracted by warm foods and unmixed wine. From the vernal equinox to the rising of the Pleiades phlegm and the sweet sera of the blood increase; food should be flavoured with sharp and pungent vegetable juices, and plenty of exercise should be taken. From the setting of the Pleiades onwards yellow bile and bitter sera in the blood increase until the summer solstice. For these take sweet things that will relax the bowels. From the summer solstice black bile increases until the autumn equinox. Take cold and sweet-smelling food. From the autumn equinox until the setting of the Pleiades, phlegm and the fine sera of the blood increase. Reduce the amount of phlegm by taking the most pungent and stinging foods, and do not take much exercise. From the setting of the Pleiades until the winter solstice take the most astringent foods, drink the sweetest wine, also fatty foods. Take large amounts of exercise.

Special limitations are placed on sexual intercourse. In the first and second of these periods it is encouraged; in the third it is to be reduced to a minimum, and likewise in the fourth, according to a handbook. In the fifth period there is to be abstention, and for the last period it is not mentioned at all.

The material of these seasonal constitutions and their effect, and of the regimen prescribed, is much the same as may be found in the dietetic books of the Hippocratic Corpus, along with *The Nature of Man* and parts of *Airs, Waters, Places* and *Epidemics*. The *Letter* is a summary document, and its purpose is not at once obvious. Medical hints for the formidable Antigonus would come more abundantly and naturally from a physician resident at court. But when we think of later ages of patronage, not only in Greek times, we can see in the *Letter* something more like an advertisement for the activities of Diocles, and a request for royal support and approval in the age of Hellenistic kings. The Macedonian kings who controlled Athens, sometimes more strictly, sometimes less, could act as patrons of medicine and other kinds of learning, but needed the advice of experts. It is surely in the role of an expert that Diocles presents himself, and the *Letter* is a form of dedication.

Diocles is known to have been a member of Aristotle's school, the Peripatetics, which, under such figures as Theophrastus and Strato, was the principal school of science in Greek lands before the new development in Alexandria.[355] Under the influence of Philistion, Plato and Aristotle accepted a form of Empedocles' theory of elements and also the theory of *pneuma*, which was dominant in so much medical speculation. This too is the origin of Aristotle's belief in the mental activity of the heart, where he is retrograde in comparison with Plato and some of the Hippocratics. In view of Aristotle's wide interests, not least in zoology and medicine (according to Plutarch he inculcated a love of medicine in his pupil Alexander the Great), it is curious that his contributions to human anatomy and physiology are so slight – apart from some good descriptions of certain organs. Nevertheless his general concepts had immense influence on later generations, not least upon one of the last great medical writers, Galen. The continuing interest of the Peripatetics in medicine as well as in biology is shown in the many medical questions raised in the pseudo-Aristotelian *Problems*, recognized now as a product of the Peripatetics rather than of Aristotle himself. The questions are often the same as those that occupied the Hippocratics.

The last figure of note before the Alexandrians is Praxagoras of Cos, who was a little younger than Diocles.[356] Very little remains of his actual words, but the titles of his works preserved in Galen and elsewhere are *Physics* (Φυσικά), in at least two books, *Anatomy* ('Ανατομή), in several books, *Diseases* (Περὶ νούσων), in at least three books, *On Foreign Diseases* (Περὶ τῶν ἀλλοτρίων παθῶν), in at least two books, *Contributory Signs* (Τὰ συνεδρεύοντα) (those which help to establish a diagnosis), in two books, *Supervening Maladies* (Τὰ ἐπιγινόμενα), on additional disorders which make a worse prognosis for the original illness, *On Treatments* (Περὶ θεραπειῶν), in at least four books, and *Causes, Illnesses and Treatments* (Αἴτια, πάθη, θεραπεῖαι), in several books; also probably a book called *On Humours* (Περὶ χυμῶν).

By his doctrine he was later classified as a Dogmatist by Galen and others; this label was also given to Diocles. The meaning is that he taught positive and definite doctrines, showing a cast of mind that was condemned under this name by the Sceptics of Plato's Academy and later in Alexandria by the Empiric sect of medical theorists.[357] The same title would have been deserved by many earlier physicians and by most nature philosophers, who were too confident that mere reason could reach truth unaided by continual testing and observation.

In physiology Praxagoras claimed to have distinguished more humours than the traditional four, namely the sweet, the uniformly mixed, the glassy, the acid, the nitrous, the salty, the bitter, the leek-green, the yolk-coloured, the corrosive and the clotting. This multiplication was certainly an advance on the simple classification of earlier writers; under the action of heat they might account more exactly for observed fact. Praxagoras and his school are known to have studied closely the relation between foods that they knew and the humours in which they believed. In the normal way nourishment turned into blood, but in pathological conditions it turned into humours, which they regarded as morbid. The various humours developed when the innate heat of the body was not normal in amount. But the heat itself had to be maintained by an intake of food having the right qualities for the nature and constitution of the feeding animal. This doctrine is a continuation of the one found in *Ancient Medicine*. Praxagoras, indeed, was regarded as the physician who had perfected dietetics. Furthermore, he did not consider that a

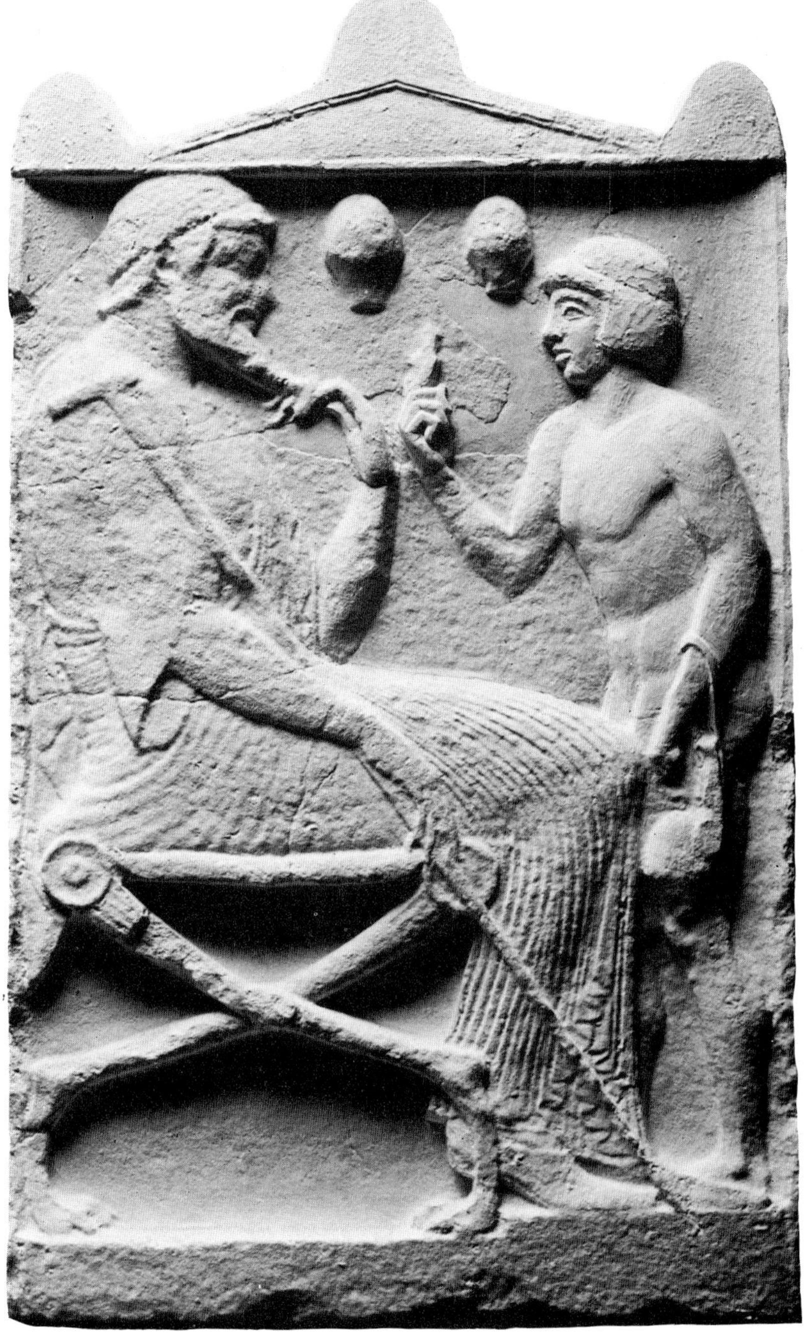

8 Fifth-century BC tombstone of a physician and boy attendant. The physician is seated on a folding stool holding his long staff of office and stroking his beard, the boy (much restored) carries an aryballos of oil. Two vessels for cupping are shown between the figures. Such cups, made of bronze, have been excavated from a number of sites (see pp. 184–5; Antikenmuseum, Basel).

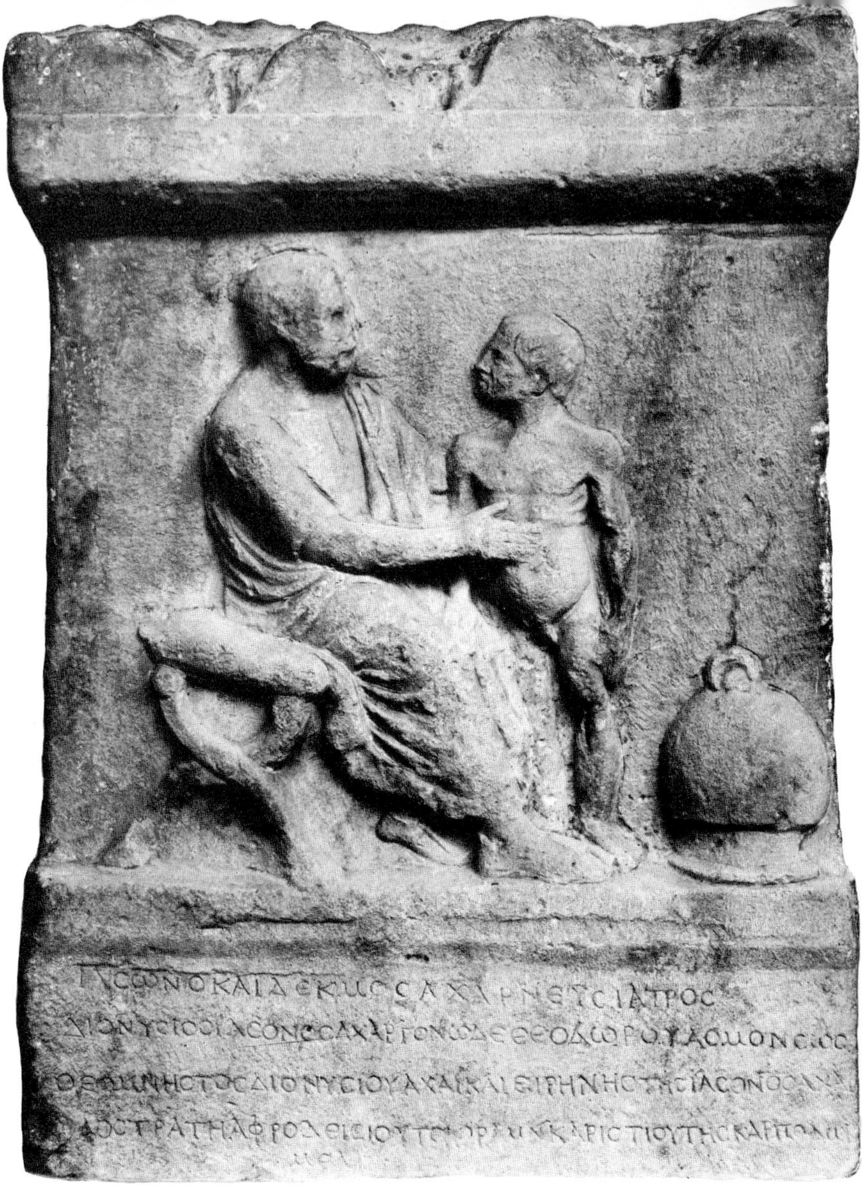

9 The tombstone of Jason, an Athenian physician of the early second century AD. He is shown seated on a folding stool and examining a young boy who appears to be rather undernourished. The object to the right is a much enlarged cupping vessel (*cf.* Plate 8) (British Museum, London).

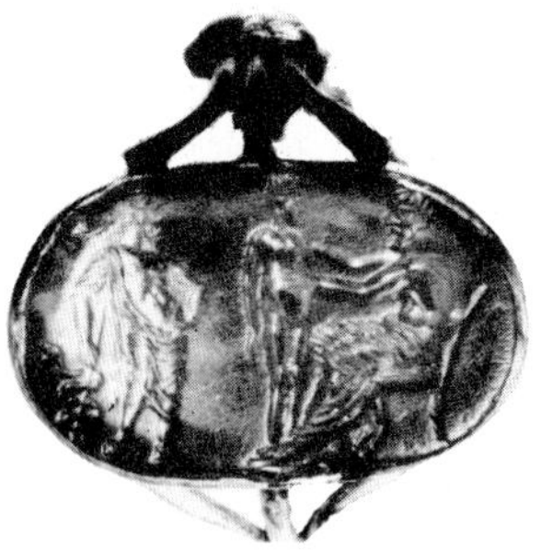

10 This fine classical gemstone shows a seated physician examining a young male patient while Asclepius looks on. A ring set with such a stone may well have belonged to a practising physician (British Museum, London).

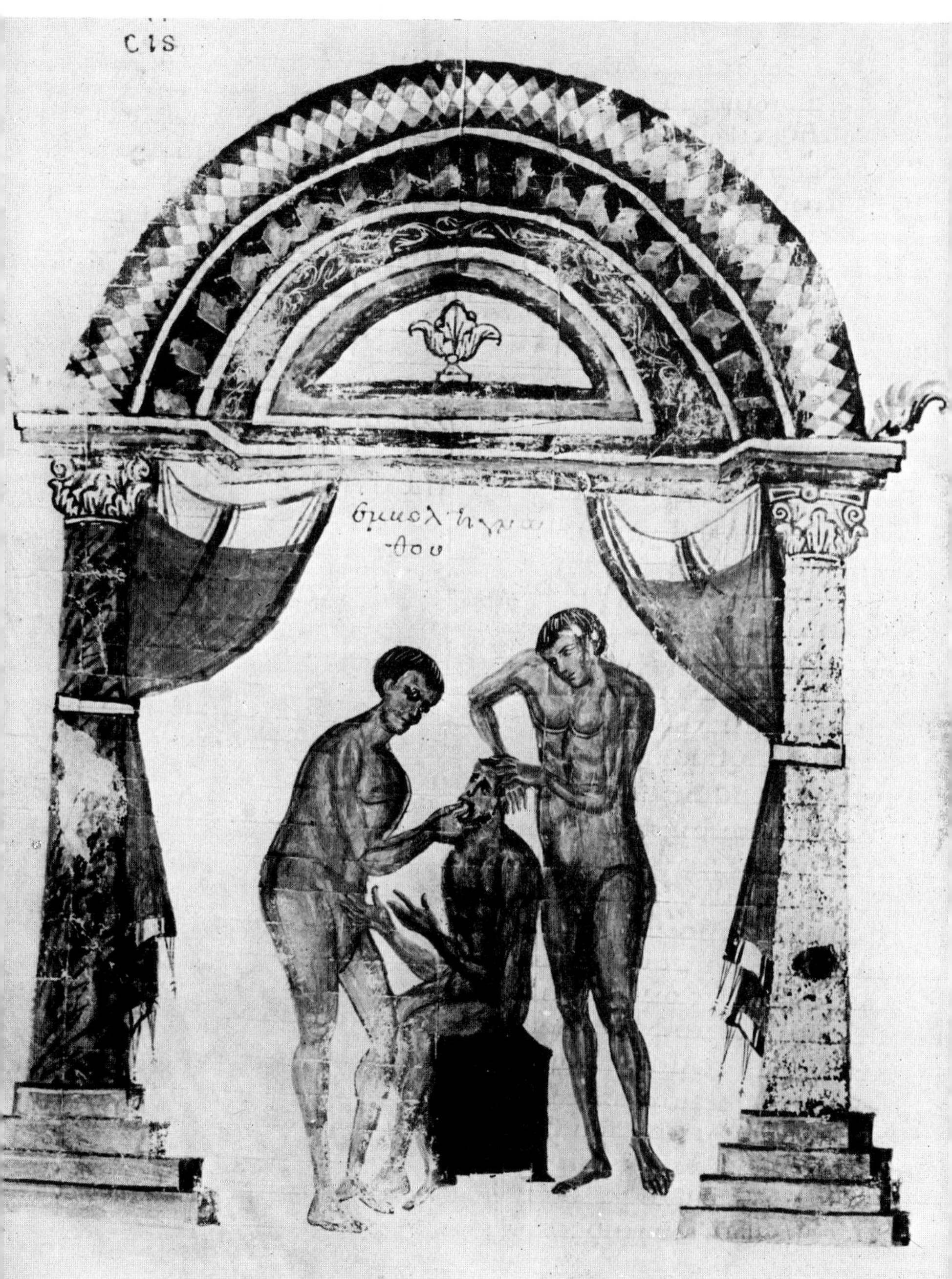

11 Ms. illustration of the reduction of a jaw (Ms. Laur. Plut. 74.7, fol. 198v, commentary by Apollonius of Kition on Hippocrates; Bibliotheca Medicea-Laurenziana, Florence).

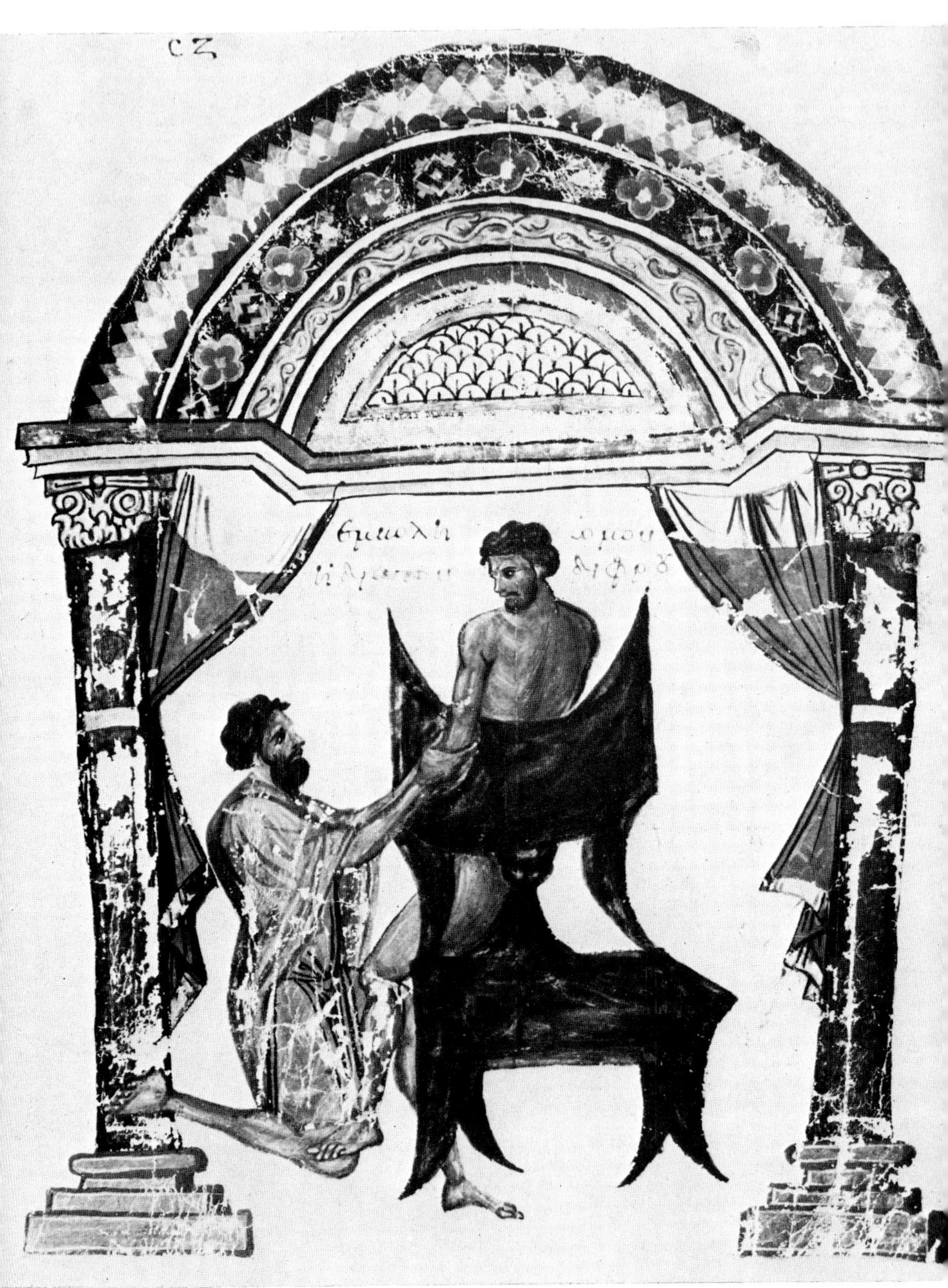

12 Reduction of the shoulder over the back of a chair (Ms. Laur. Plut. 74.7, fol. 190, commentary by Apollonius of Kition on Hippocrates; Bibliotheca Medicea-Laurenziana, Florence).

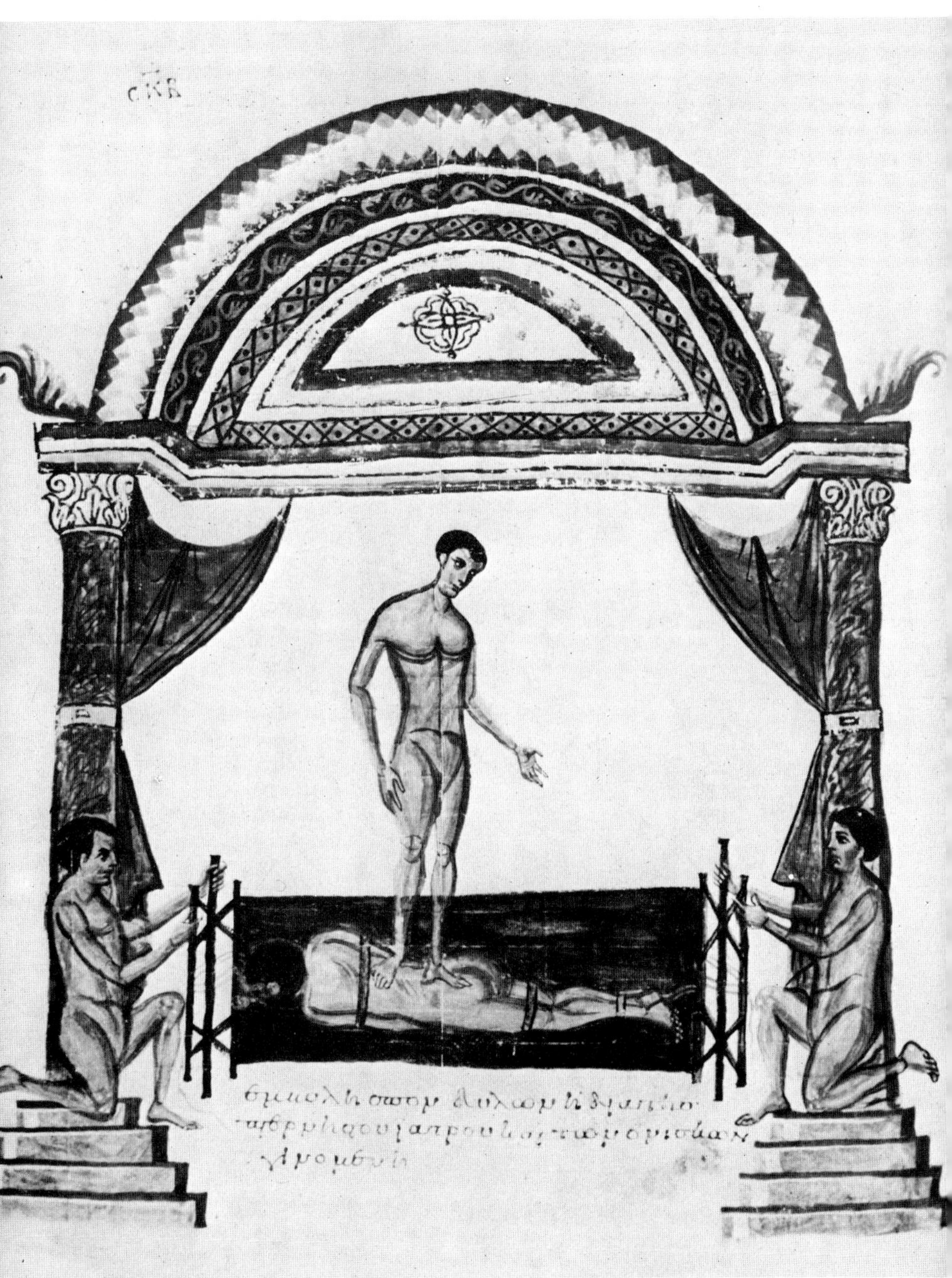

13 Reduction of the vertebrae by traction and windlass and a man standing on the patient's back (Ms. Laur. Plut. 74.7, fol. 203v, commentary by Apollonius of Kition on Hippocrates; Bibliotheca Medicea-Laurenziana, Florence).

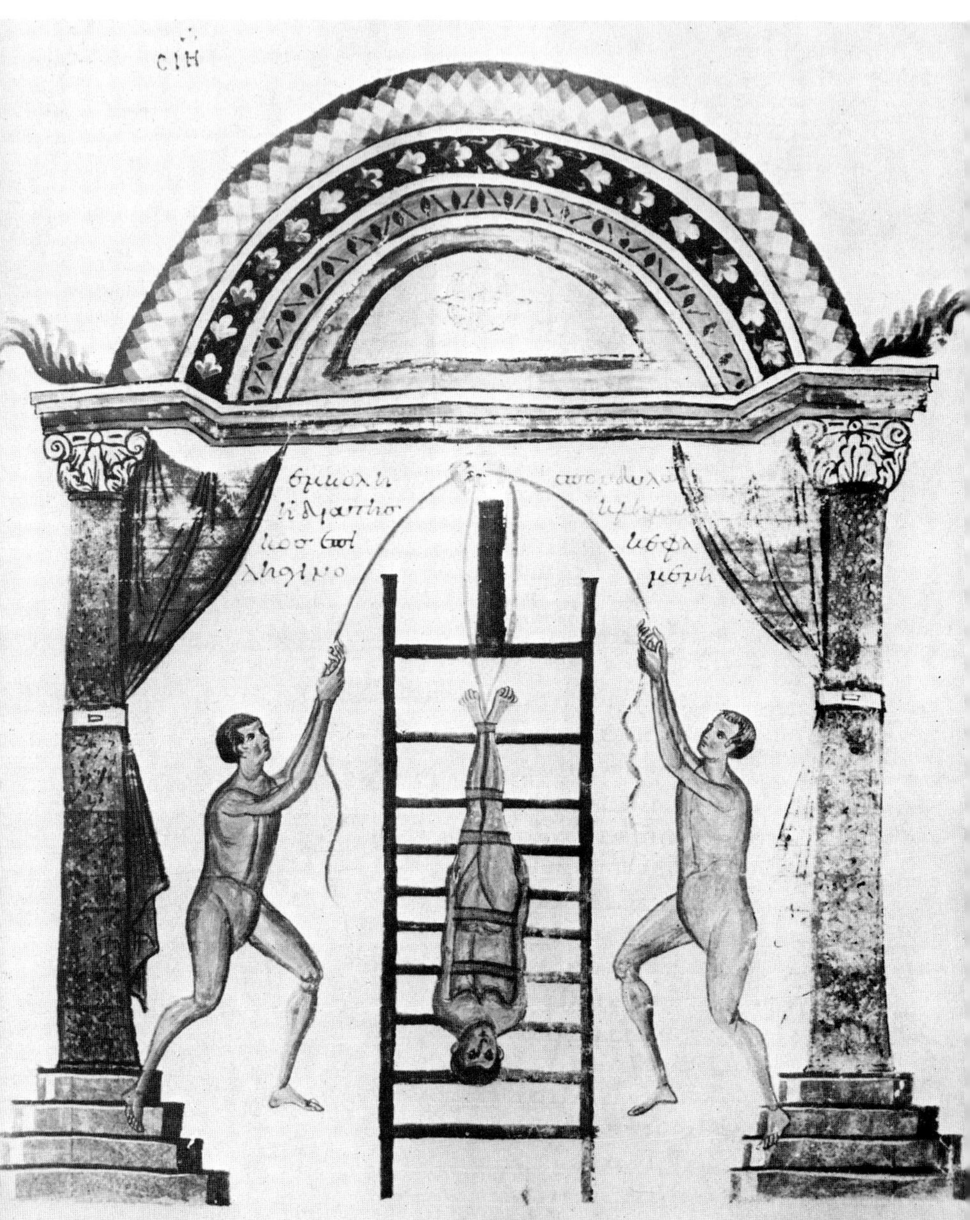

14 Reduction of the vertebrae by succussion on a ladder (Ms. Laur. Plut. 74.7, fol. 200, commentary by Apollonius of Kition on Hippocrates; Bibliotheca Medicea-Laurenziana, Florence).

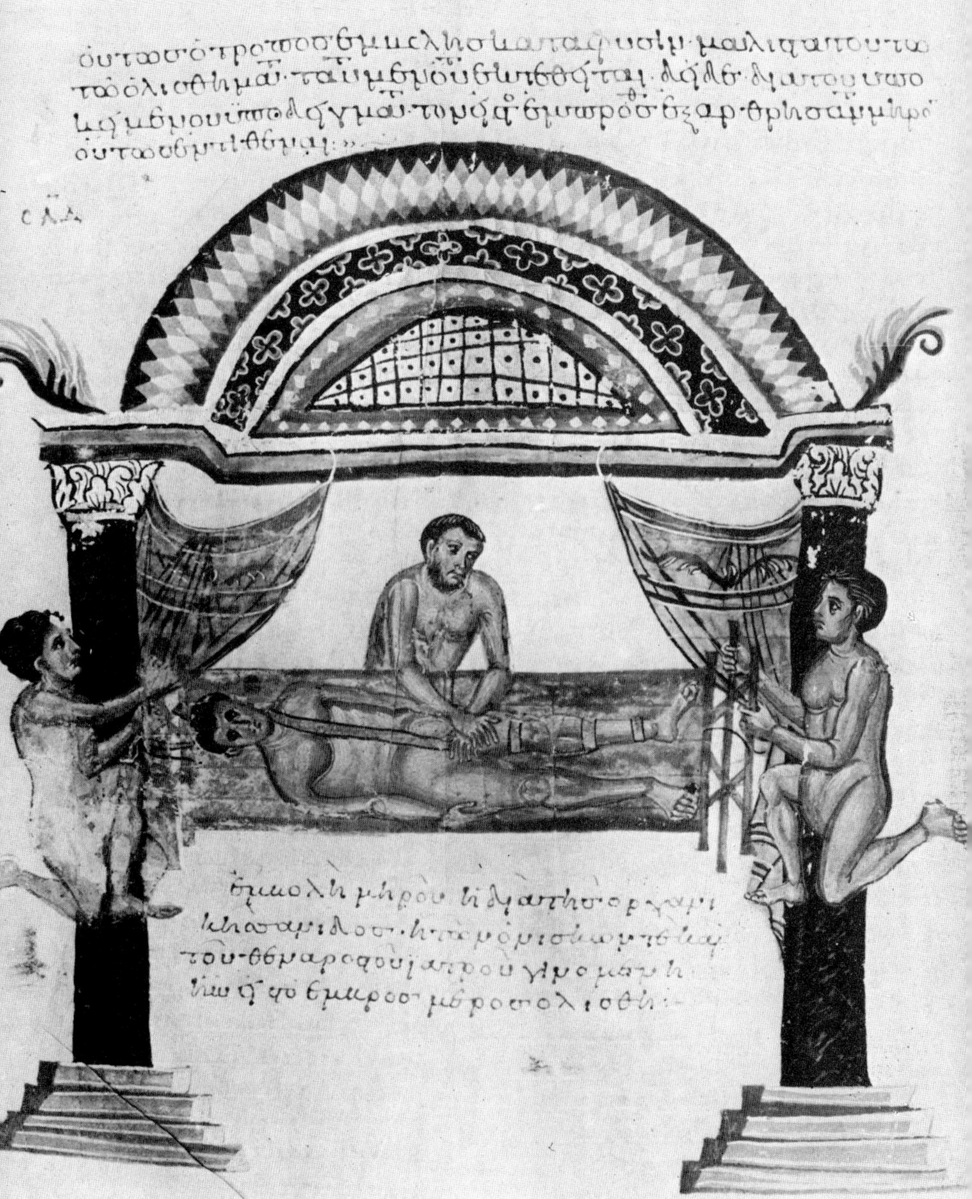

15 Reduction of the femur by traction and a socket windlass (Ms. Laur. Plut. 74.7, fol. 222v, commentary by Apollonius of Kition on Hippocrates; Bibliotheca Medicea-Laurenziana, Florence).

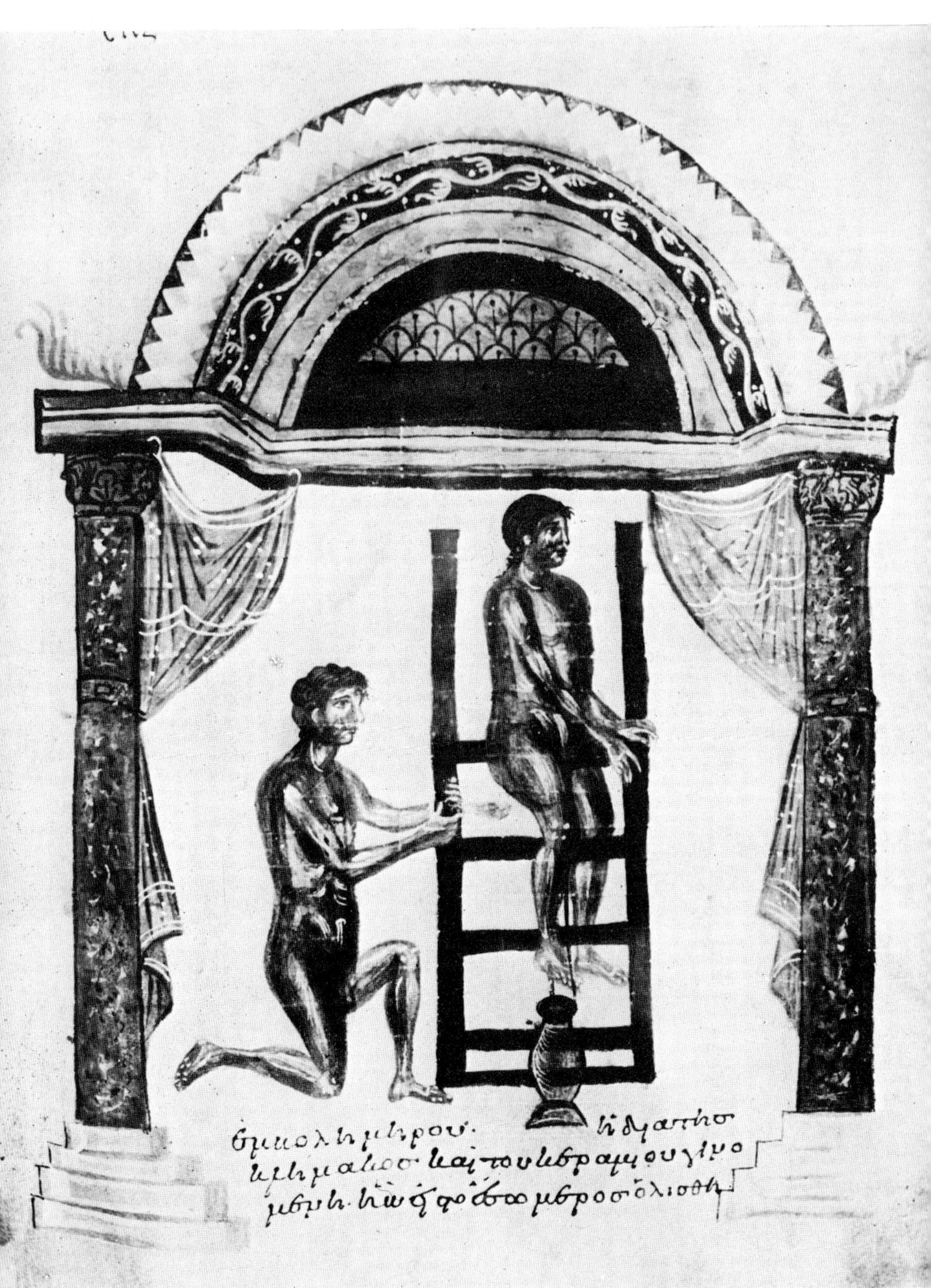

16 Reduction of the femur by use of a ladder and weights (Ms. Laur. Plut. 74.7, fol. 209, commentary by Apollonius of Kition on Hippocrates; Bibliotheca Medicea-Laurenziana, Florence).

general enquiry into the qualities and effects of a certain food was enough; general dietetics must be supplemented by individual, for what will benefit one man will harm another, so different are the natures of men. On the effects of phlegm and bile Praxagoras held the same views as earlier physicians. He also made a thorough enquiry into cures by hunger.[358]

Other features of his physiology are to be explained by his beliefs about anatomy. He was one of the earliest to distinguish clearly between veins and arteries and between their contents, though by no means in our fashion. He held that the arteries originate in the heart and are filled with *pneuma*, not with blood. Near the heart they are rather large ducts, but further out they become divided into increasingly narrow vessels, until, when their walls meet with no hollow bore or lumen any longer between them, they become *neura*. The word *neura* was still commonly used for tendons, which were known to move bones in muscular action; but since *pneuma* was thought to be the originator of movement, it seems that here it has begun to be used for nerves as they came to be distinguished. From this report in Galen, who knew the true function of the tissues that we call nerves, it appears that Praxagoras was one of the first to distinguish them, though this line of research was carried much further and to much more definite results by the Alexandrians. Praxagoras thus believed that arteries and nerves were part of the same ramifying system, though Galen exaggerates when he berates Praxagoras for asserting that nerves originate in the heart.[359] Yet the difficulty remains of connecting the functions of the nerves, as they were beginning to be known, with that of the heart as the Western tradition of medicine believed it to be. The white *neura* with no lumen have to carry the vivifying *pneuma* to the extremities. The veins on the other hand carried blood from which the flesh was formed, but this had bubbles in it.

Praxagoras conceived the *pneuma* as the denser part of the surrounding air; he did not, as Aristotle did, believe in innate *pneuma*. Thus for him breathing was a direct nourishing of the soul, which was more precisely the *pneuma* in the heart. This should imply that there was a direct connection from the lungs to the heart, carrying *pneuma*. But the *pneuma* in the heart included also other *pneuma*, collected from the body partly by general respiration of the entire body, for which an intake through the pores would be necessary, and partly from the blood in the veins. In this respect his theory of pulses is particularly important.[360]

He defined pulse (σφυγμός) as a movement of the arteries, but only the natural or normal movement as distinct from morbid tremors (παλμός, τρόμος and σπασμός). Like other earlier writers, he believed that the arteries did not owe their pulsation mechanically to the heart, but attributed it to bubbles derived from the blood in the veins.[361] These bubbles passed through the heart and entered the arteries, but the blood did not. Released into the arteries, they provoked pulsing in their walls. The contractions of this pulsing burst the bubbles, which thus released into the arteries *pneuma* from the body added to that brought by inspiration. When the blood was normal the bubbling process was steady, but when it contained morbid humours the bubbling was irregular. Thus regular and natural pulsation of the arteries indicated healthy blood in the veins, and irregular pulsation blood contaminated with these humours.[362]

These methods of argument were intended by Praxagoras to guide discovery to the original cause of a disease, which was distinct from all the manifestations by which it was known, including its variation from one individual to another. His therapy attempted to reach this original cause. He also developed a strong interest in surgery. He did not hesitate to cut off the uvula completely in some cases where it was inflamed. In a case of hernia where an intestinal loop slipped down into the scrotum, he opened the abdomen, cut the intestines, removed faecal matter, and sewed everything together again. This exceptional operation was not admired. From his surgery he appears to have learned more anatomy, though he still lived before the age of regular dissection.[363]

Of his pupils, Phylotimus, Plistonicus and Xenophon followed closely in his footsteps and originated nothing new, but Herophilus, who disagreed with him, is one of the great names of the next phase of medicine.[364]

CHAPTER VI

THE ALEXANDRIAN SCHOOL OF MEDICINE

During the period treated in the last chapter comparatively little was added to the knowledge, thought and methods which are found in the Hippocratic books and which are due to the older schools of medicine. To judge from the scanty remains of this period it was an age of consolidation and refinement, but, in spite of the Aristotelian and Peripatetic influence, hardly one of discovery in medical science. It is still uncertain whether any advance was made then in human anatomy by direct observation.[365] The Alexandrian age in its opening years, however, was very different; for to this phase belong the most important known advances on previous knowledge of anatomical and physiological fact that were ever made in the ancient world. This progress was part of the whole growth of Alexandrian science in the Museum, or Royal Academy, established by Ptolemy I, and it is likely that the other sciences had a stimulating effect on medicine, if only by example, as in modern times.[366] Thus Alexandrian medicine can be regarded as a slight foretaste of the medical discoveries made in the sixteenth and later centuries of our own civilization. But the impetus of discovery did not last long, for reasons which will be set forth.

Among the scholars and scientists that Ptolemy collected from Athens and other Greek cities were the two great physicians Herophilus of Chalcedon, a pupil of Praxagoras, and Erasistratus of Iulis on the island of Ceos, who appears to have studied at Athens with the Peripatetics before learning medicine on Cos.[367] They made their advances by beginning the regular practice of dissection, and some remarks on this subject are necessary before we begin to explore their discoveries and their doctrines.

Diocles had already written a book, *On Anatomy*, which was the first to be concerned entirely with the subject; this book, as we noted, has perished. The literal meaning of ἀνατομή is simply 'cutting up' or 'dissection', and it has been argued that, although there was no regular practice of dissection before the Alexandrians, the decisive change in the way of regarding the human body, and in the dogma concerning it, occurred early in the history of the Peripatetic school, to which Diocles was attached. This would explain Galen's observation, in his historical account of anatomy, that books on the subject were first written by Diocles and after him by a few of the ancient physicians.[368] Before the time of Diocles the ancient and popular belief that the dead body still has some awareness of the things that happen to it, and therefore an absolute right to be buried intact and undisturbed, had forbidden all interference with corpses.[369] Even in the Hippocratic age, therefore, knowledge of the shape, position and interrelation of the internal organs had depended at most on unobserved investigation of strangers' bodies casually found, and on the analogies provided by cutting up animal bodies in butchery or sacrifice, both of which were used to supplement information gained by external palpation of the living body.[370]

The changed attitude to dissection among learned men and philosophers, but not among the uneducated, was due to philosophical teaching which took practical effect not long after Aristotle's death.[371] First Plato had taught that the soul was an independent and immortal being which during earthly life carried the body as a mere envelope and instrument to be discarded at death. Then Aristotle declared that the soul, though not separable and immortal, constituted the purpose and value of the whole organism, implying that after death there was no more than a physical frame without feelings or rights.[372] From this position it was no long step to claiming that the dead body could justly be used for dissection and anatomical study. So far as the dead body could provide it, knowledge by direct inspection and no longer by indirect means could now be pursued among the learned when favourable circumstances arose.

This effect of philosophy on medical science was a renewal in more precise form of the earlier effect produced on medicine by pre-Socratic speculation on nature. It was brought about paradoxically by the new content that Socrates had given to philosophy when he abandoned inquiry into nature and concerned himself only with the soul. Thus from the end of the fourth century philosophy caused as great a change in medical science as it did in the physician's attitude to his patients.

Celsus, writing under the Roman Empire, is one authority for this attitude to dissection.[373] A further stage in the development, and one which was confined to Alexandria, was vivisection of human beings, which Celsus even more emphatically attests. In the introduction to his book *De Medicina* he argues that Herophilus and Erasistratus discovered yet more about the internal organs by laying open men when they were still alive. The subjects of vivisection were criminals received out of prison from the kings, and Celsus denies that it is cruel to torture a handful of criminals in pursuit of remedies for innocent people of all future ages.[374] Tertullian in the course of his Christian apologetics denounces 'the physician or butcher who cuts up six hundred bodies in order to investigate nature, who allows himself to hate mankind'. He calls this kind of death 'not natural but made unnatural through the violence of dissection'.[375] On this subject no Greek sources seem to have been preserved. The account of Celsus has been denied as often as it has been accepted by historians, both of manners and customs and of medicine.[376] In our time the mere cruelty of the practice no longer makes it incredible, as it did to our grandfathers. What the benefit to medicine may have been it is not for a layman to determine. But if it did benefit medicine it still could not be defended by the philosophical argument used in support of the dissection of corpses. In spite of his fame, Herophilus left few writings. Apart from a commentary on the Hippocratic *Prognostic*, those reported by Galen are *Anatomy* (*'Ανατομικά*), in three books, *On the Eyes* (*Περὶ ὀφθαλμῶν*), *Midwifery* (*Μαιωτικόν*), *Pulses* (*Περὶ σφυγμῶν*), *A Treatise on Therapy* (*Θεραπευτικὴ πραγματεία*), *Regimen* (*Διαιτητικόν*) and *Against Common Opinions*[377] (*Πρὸς τὰς κοὶνας δόξας*). No doubt he was too busy as surgeon, physician and medical scientist to write more. Galen preserves a number of quotations, however, and makes some summaries or other references.

According to Galen, at the beginning of the third book of his *Anatomy* Herophilus mentions two *orcheis* set slantwise on either side of the womb.[378] *Orcheis* is the normal word for the testicles in males; here it clearly means the ovaries. The two female *orcheis* or ovaries are described as not in one scrotum like the male testicles but separated, each being enclosed in a fine membraneous envelope. They are small and flat like glands, sinewy in their envelope but solid in their flesh as in males. In mares they are large and attached to the womb by many membranes and by a vein and an artery running to them from the womb. They are interconnected by a vein and artery running from each of them to the main vein and artery attaching the other to the womb. The channels for the seed are not very conspicuous but are attached to the outer part of the womb. They run from the ovaries to the fleshy part of the neck of the bladder, as in the male, being thin and crooked in front where they touch the ischial bones. In the male the seminal vessels come to an end as they penetrate the penis. But the varicose channel is not found in the female.

Galen comments that Herophilus makes these female vessels too like the male: they are not so small and they do not run to the neck of the bladder.[379] That is to say, the female's Fallopian tubes are much less like the *vesiculae seminales*, especially in position, than Herophilus says, even though he admits differences. But to have noted the Fallopian tubes at all was an important advance in anatomy. The reference to mares suggests an interest in comparative anatomy, rather than the use of animal anatomy for analogical inference, since Herophilus had access to human corpses, unlike later writers who were forced back upon the animal analogy. But the general plan of the genital organs differs little from one mammal to another. Herophilus also compares the womb to a semicircle: the semicircular curve would be below the diameter.[380] In the abdomen Herophilus discovered a vessel intended for nourishing the intestines, without, as he says, passing into the liver, as all the other vessels in this region do; it terminated in bodies like glands. His name, δωδεκαδάκτυλον, 'twelve finger-widths' long', for the passage from the stomach to the beginning of the intestines is still preserved in the Latin rendering as *duodenum*.[381]

Herophilus made a beginning at least in discovering the salivary glands at the root of the tongue, the glands from the stomach which discharge into the entrails, the discharge of bile from the liver and another form of moisture from other glands which is like saliva.[382] Galen remarks that anatomists since Herophilus and Eudemus had done much research on these glands.[383] Concerning the vascular system Herophilus had a more sensible doctrine than those who believed that the arteries carried no blood but only *pneuma*. Galen says that, like Praxagoras, Phylotimus, Diocles and others, he held that *pneuma* was not propelled through the vessels, but drawn through them by attraction, and did not come from the heart only; also that he saw that the arteries were full of blood, for the diastole of the arteries had its source in the heart, which drove the blood.[384] Herophilus also noticed how much thicker the walls of the arteries were than those of the veins, indeed six times as thick, though no inference of his from this fact as to their function has been preserved. He saw that the walls of arteries were loose and empty in death, but also how widely separated they were in life.[385] In fact in earlier writers the original reason for assuming that the arteries carried only *pneuma* had been that those near the heart were found to be empty of blood at death.

Thus it was natural that Herophilus should have been the founder of sphygmology, the systematic study of the pulse, even if others had paid some attention to the subject before him. Praxagoras had supposed that the arteries had an independent power of pulsation.[386] Herophilus denied this independence; he seems to have believed that there was some sympathy of the arteries with the heart, but still thought that arterial pulsation was an action of the arteries themselves.[387] He cannot have considered the fluid content either of the heart or of the arteries as essential to the process of pulsation. But at least he was right in saying that abnormal tremors and spasms in the arteries were not different in kind from regular pulsation, but only in magnitude. He established that the veins did not originate in the liver, but could not decide where they did originate.[388] Indeed he seems to have paid relatively little attention to the veins, so that he could never have conceived a theory of circulation.

Herophilus also made a careful study of the liver.[389] He distinguished the bile ducts from the portal veins, though he may not have understood their importance. He was a pioneer in comparative anatomy, for he compared the human liver with the hare's, and noted that all blooded animals, as Aristotle called vertebrates, had livers, though they varied in their size and structure and in the number of lobes. He found some variation in these even in man.

In the lungs he observed a vein which was like an artery, by which he must have meant that it had a thick wall and pulsated.[390] This would be the pulmonary artery through which blood, in this case of the venous kind, is pumped into the pulmonary vessels for oxygenation. But how much he understood of its nature and function is not certain; he should surely have noticed also the pulmonary vein which returns the oxygenated blood to the heart. Herophilus is credited with the first attempt to count the frequency of the pulse against the outflow of a water-clock filled with a definite amount of water, and is said to have settled the natural frequency of the pulse for various ages of human life.[391] But it is not known whether these measurements were ever taken again.

The best work of Herophilus, however, was in his investigation of the nervous system. He maintained that all the *neura*, white cords resembling sinews but conveying sensations which ran about the body below the head, originated either from the fourth ventricle of the brain, by the cerebellum (*παρεγκέφαλις*), or from the spinal marrow. They were supplied with *pneuma* from a ventricle (*κοιλία*) in the brain which was of a notable size and received the psychic *pneuma* made in the lateral ventricles further forward. This ventricle was large, and the channels running into it from the forward ventricles were also very large.[392] In terms of modern anatomy, Herophilus is here speaking of the third ventricle, situated in the thalamencephalon and connected in fact by two forward channels with the lateral ventricles.

Close by this channel, he said, was the insertion of the cerebellum into the brain. Galen, who reproduces this description, would have preferred to call the fourth ventricle, which lies further back, sovereign, no doubt because it is nearer to the central canal of the spinal cord.[393] Herophilus may not have distinguished the fourth ventricle clearly enough from the third in his writing, as Erasistratus did. The *pneuma* in these ventricles is replaced in modern anatomy by the cerebro-spinal fluid.

Herophilus applied the epithet *chorioeides*, 'like the chorion', to the meninges, because he thought of them as like the two membranes, chorion and amnion, which envelope the foetus in the womb. This way of thought survives in the Latin expressions *pia mater* and *dura mater* which we still use. In his neurology of the body Herophilus remarked that some paralyses destroyed sensation only, others voluntary movement only, and others again both. But he left the cause of these differences unexplained and Galen used this as an example of the shortcomings of mere anatomy.[394] Herophilus appears to have identified sensory nerves clearly enough, but may have failed to define motor nerves properly, or to distinguish them always from sinews. In his time it was naturally unknown what areas of the brain controlled what actions or received what stimuli. For him nerves were still channels for the movement of *pneuma*.[395] *Pneuma* as vital air was one of the most long-lived notions in medicine, like the humours.[396] Galen uses the term 'psychic *pneuma*' in his account of Herophilus on the brain; in his time this finer grade of *pneuma* was distinguished from merely vital *pneuma* elsewhere.[397]

In the matter of obstetrics Herophilus, along with Hippocrates and Erasistratus, is denounced by Tertullian for using an instrument called ἐμβρυοσφάκτης, a form of bronze rod for killing a live infant, no doubt in cases of very difficult birth.[398] A fragment of Herophilus' handbook of obstetrics mentions various difficult positions of the embryo in presentation, and even birth with the membrane still unbroken.[399] He was celebrated as an obstetrician. His account of respiration is taken over from Praxagoras with little change.

Such is the scanty material in extract and allusion for our knowledge of Herophilus. For Erasistratus, his contemporary and rival at Alexandria, we are rather better served. His works as named in ancient sources are the following: his main work in anatomy, called *Divisions* (*Διαιρέσεις*), in two books, written in old age; the *General Treatise* (*Περὶ τῶν καθόλου λόγων*), in at least two books; *Hints on Health* (*Ὑγιεινά*), in two books; *Fevers* (*Περὶ πυρετῶν*), in three books; *On Drawing Blood* (*Περὶ αἵματος ἀναγωγῆς*), in two books; *On Causes* (*Περὶ αἰτιῶν*); *On Diseases of the Intestines* (*Περὶ τῶν κατὰ τὴν κοιλίαν παθῶν*); *On Paralysis* (*Περὶ παραλύσεως*), in two books; *On Gout* (*Περὶ ποδάγρας*); *On Dropsy* (*Περὶ ὕδρωπος*), *On Powers and Lethal Substances* (*Περὶ δυνάμεων καὶ θανασίμων*), apparently on the effects and the dangers of various drugs; and his *Cookery Book* (*Ὀψαρτυτικά*).[400]

Erasistratus set his medical opinions more definitely in the context of general science. As we saw, some of the Hippocratics had done this before him, if pre-Socratic nature philosophy can be called science. But Erasistratus took account of Democritus' atomic theory, which comes nearer to science as we understand it, and also of Peripatetic science from Aristotle's time onward. The Democritean theory of atoms does not appear in known medical writing before him. His strictly medical training, which followed his stay in Athens with the Peripatetics, was given to him for a short time on Cos with the school of Praxagoras, and for a longer time at Alexandria, where Chrysippus the younger, of the rival Cnidian school, had founded a new school of his own.[401] To Chrysippus he owed various doctrines, methods and attitudes which were different from those of most physicians. For the last years of his stay in Alexandria he abandoned medical practice for the pursuit of anatomy and physiology as sciences. He may be called the first known professor of anatomy and physiology.

Galen's comments on his general attitude in medicine are interesting. While nearly all writers, he says, including the Peripatetics, praise nature as a craftsman, Erasistratus and his followers do not agree at all. Erasistratus claims that the Peripatetics are entirely wrong concerning nature. He asserts one thing in common with them, that nature does everything for some purpose and nothing to no purpose; yet he does not keep to this principle everywhere, for he says that there is no purpose in the spleen, in the epiplöon and in many other organs.[402] Modern physiologists might approve of Erasistratus for not holding a strict teleology in the manner of Aristotle and, long after him, of Galen; but if Galen's report is correct they would say rather that Erasistratus cannot have found physiological functions for these organs. Anyway, there is always a flavour of teleology about the word 'function' in biology. In ancient philosophy it is a fact that teleology was increasingly abandoned among those Peripatetics who were scientists, so that Erasistratus may have had his doubts or qualifications while he was studying with the Peripatetics.

In anatomy Erasistratus made remarkable progress, basing himself on the predecessors mentioned and enjoying the Alexandrian licence to dissect. He carried further the investigations of Herophilus in comparative anatomy, noting the differences in the formation of the brain between man and animals.[403] He saw the importance of the different tissues in the human body, perhaps better than Galen allows. He recognized that every organ and every part of the intestines had accompanying veins, arteries and nerves, and for the whole of these systems he used the expression *τριπλοκία τῶν ἀγγείων*, 'three-fold network' or 'three-fold plaiting of vessels'.[404] 'Plaiting' would still be appropriate where nerves, veins and arteries are laid very close together. We should agree that every nerve needs its blood supply brought by arteries and drained away, with its impurities, by veins. He assumed that veins, arteries and nerves had at their extremities *lumina* so fine that they were no longer accessible to the senses and could be recognized only by the reason. All tissues were held together by this kind of plaiting, as by a rope made of three differing strands. Erasistratus more than any other ancient anatomist would have been grateful for a microscope to pursue the assumptions of his reason much further than his unaided sight took him into the recesses of histology, as we now call it.

Erasistratus described the brain more accurately than Herophilus. He distinguished the greater brain, or cerebrum (*ἐγκέφαλος*), from the lesser or cerebellum (*ἐπεγκρανίς* in his terminology, not *παρεγκεφαλίς* as in Herophilus).[405] He described the two lateral ventricles of the cerebrum as small hollows, the third ventricle as communicating with them by a cleft (our own *foramen interventriculare*) and the fourth as inside the cerebellum, connected by a channel (our *aqueductus sylvii*) to the third. Each of these parts of the brain is enclosed in membranes of skin, the λεπτὴ μήνιγξ (our *pia mater*) and the μήνιγξ παχεῖα (our *dura mater*).[406] The surface of both is mostly occupied by winding and forking structures, our 'convolutions', by which he explained the greater intelligence of man as compared to animals.[407] Like Herophilus, he conceived the ventricles as being filled during life with psychic *pneuma*, conveyed to them from the heart by the arteries. Like Herophilus again, he declared that the brain was the originating point for all the nerves. These he at first believed to spring from the *dura mater*, because he had found by experiment that incisions in the *dura mater* robbed animals of their power of movement. In old age he changed his view as a result of further experiment, saying that all nerves originated from the inner brain and that cords of the same tissue ran inwards from the organs of the special senses, hearing, sight, taste and smell.[408] In the first place he distinguished sensory from motor nerves (νεῦρα αἰσθητικά and κινητικά).[409] The nerve fibres he conceived as being composed of three strands, veins, arteries and *neura*, and nourished by the veins. At first he believed that the nerves were hollow and filled with *pneuma* and were therefore vessels, but later he recognized that they were solid, consisting of marrow of the spinal kind.[410]

Movement was carried out by the muscles, equally made up of veins, arteries and nerves. The *pneuma* reaching them enabled them to contract, that is to become broader while they reduced their length.[411] If this account is true, it is surprising that so acute an investigator did not perceive that muscles are not made of nerves, arteries and veins, even though they have them and their continued action depends on them. But ancient medicine was mostly ill-informed about muscles. The rest of Erasistratus' anatomy is best considered along with his physiology.

In physiology Erasistratus is remarkable for two innovations in general theory. He set aside the multiplication of humours that Praxagoras and his school had introduced, and was, indeed, inclined to pay very little attention to humoral theory at all.

He considered that all investigation into the origin of humours was labour lost, and never so much as mentioned black bile. But he did allow some place to morbid alteration of the chyle produced by digestion, to glutinous and chilly humours as the cause of apoplexy and paralysis, and to excess of bilious humours as the origin of jaundice – this last opinion is perfectly correct.[412] None the less he had shown the way to ending the dominance of humoral theory. Unfortunately this way was not further followed in antiquity. In Galen, for instance, the humours are still canonical.

His other innovation was to apply atomic theory and other notions of physics to the processes of physiology. He combined the Democritean doctrine of atoms and void with the doctrine of *pneuma* that came down to him from Praxagoras and his predecessors. He was determined to trace all the phenomena of the body to these natural causes, as he saw them, whose workings would often be on an invisibly small scale. He rejected all occult powers, such as that of attraction (ἕλξις), alleged by some physicians to be a cause of movement in the body's fluids, and wherever possible explained this by his principle of ἀκολουθία πρὸς τὸ κενούμενον, or 'following on into empty space', which we may conveniently translate by *horror vacui*.[413] But he still retained the idea of nature as craftsman, using foresight on behalf of living creatures to form all parts of the body in perfect fashion for their work.[414] These two strands in his thought were not really compatible, as Galen saw. Anatomy and physiology of this date were not yet troubled with useless vestigial organs such as the vermiform appendix, with their attendant inconveniences, which our own thought can explain in an evolutionary framework.

The function of the blood in nourishing individual organs was made possible by a primal vein whose ramifications were everywhere.[415] This would be our *vena cava*, conceived in a different role. The distribution of nourishment (διάδοσις) to the vessels themselves was not effected through their ends, but through their walls, obliquely to the line of flow, by a process of resorption in which the atoms of nourishment made their way by *horror vacui* through fine cavities into the venous walls. Blood brought by the veins to the brain, spinal marrow, liver, spleen and lungs passed through the veins entering these tissues to renew the substance of each.[416] To us this appears unsatisfactory because the same flux of blood, if it actually formed the tissues, would have a different product in each tissue. But Erasistratus had not our aids to histology, which would have revealed that each tissue has its characteristic cells.

Erasistratus accepted the doctrine of *pneuma* from his predecessors, even following Praxagoras' belief that the arteries held no blood but only *pneuma*, an entirely different and separate substance.[417] The contradiction of this doctrine which bleeding arteries implied he explained by using *horror vacui* in a peculiar way. When an artery was wounded, he supposed that *pneuma* rushed out of it, leaving something like a vacuum, which was filled by blood from the neighbouring veins entering through fine capillaries (συναναστομώσεις), which in ordinary circumstances were closed. This transfer of blood he called παρέμπτωσις, 'transfusion sideways'.[418]

The doctrine of *pneuma* also caused difficulties in his account of the heart, since he regarded this organ as the distributor both of blood and of *pneuma*, of the blood through the veins, of the *pneuma* through the arteries. Thus the left ventricle of the heart was the gathering place of *pneuma* only, and the right ventricle of blood only. With every diastole of the heart these different substances were sucked into their separate ventricles, and with every systole blood was driven into the lungs and *pneuma* through the aorta into the arterial system.[419] Erasistratus thus went some way towards linking the two flows which we call the pulmonary and the systemic circulations. But as he never ceased to believe that the arteries contained only *pneuma* he was barred from anticipating Harvey in understanding that the same blood passed in different states through arteries and veins. Indeed it is not clear how he believed that blood made its way about the body, if it went from the right ventricle to the lungs and then back to the heart without entering the left ventricle. The left ventricle and the aorta are indeed the only way out into the system, but this way was reserved for the *pneuma* and so blood was not allowed to take it.

Nutrition was rightly connected by Erasistratus with the movement of the blood. The moist and the dry elements in food were mixed in the mouth, and then reached the stomach via the gullet. He knew of the service of the epiglottis in checking the descent of food into the windpipe, and thus corrected the mistake of older writers who had believed that drinks reached the lungs.[420] In the stomach were two different layers of muscle, the fibres of the inner one arranged in a ring pattern and those of the outer one longitudinally. These muscles worked the food over by peristaltic action, assisted by *pneuma* drawn in from the stomachic arteries. For this reason the digestive power of the stomach was impaired in fever, since in this state the *pneuma* was blocked in its movement by intruding blood and could not reach the stomach.[421] Erasistratus rejected the opinion of Diocles and Plistonicus that the contents of the stomach underwent a sort of fermentation or putrefaction, and also the view of Aristotle and the older physicians that they were in some sense cooked by the heat.[422] His whole account of digestion in the stomach was too much influenced by the crudely physical notions of the atomists, who saw all processes in terms of moving and squeezing, of blocking and repulsion. Its tendency was directly against any approach to a chemical theory of digestion, as we should call it.

From the stomach and intestine the liquefied food was forced by the pressure of the stomach into the blood vessels and driven as far as the liver, which converted it into blood – how, Erasistratus never explained.[423] Here again we are reminded of a process like the spreading of steam from a boiler through a system of pipes. While the bilious components were filtered out and carried to the gall-bladder, the purified blood passed from the liver into the *vena cava* and the heart. If the bile was stopped from flowing through the proper duct into the gall-bladder, jaundice resulted; this is correct.[424] If the veins of the liver were stopped by its hardening, so that they took in only the watery element of the chyle, the result was dropsy.[425] The excess of fluid reached the kidneys and so, by *horror vacui*, the bladder.[426] The veins absorbed nourishment by a process that Erasistratus called ἀνάδοσις, but no such absorption was effected by the arteries, which were nourished by veins in their own thickness – a neat suggestion within the theory, given the greater thickness of the arteries.[427] Digestion went better in sleep because there was not then any voluntary movement and pulses were slower. Such questions as the origin of humours Erasistratus excluded from medicine and assigned to the natural sciences.[428] This is odd in a man who admitted such remoter forms of thought as atomism and theories of mechanical movement into his own science from physics. Here again he seems to have had a bias against the kind of inquiry that eventually resulted in chemistry.

The process of nutrition and growth he saw as one of the addition of new parts to those that were already there, as new pieces are woven on to a net, a rope or a sack. This was balanced by a continual loss of matter, a point which Erasistratus tried to establish by experiment. Some of the loss was by common excretion, but some occurred by theoretically assumed but invisible exhalation (ἀποφορὰ κατὰ τὸ λόγῳ θεωρητόν).[429] This doctrine and its formulation he had from Aegimius of Elis.[430] To counteract the loss, nature gave living creatures appetites to take in matter and *pneuma* to work on it.[431]

Erasistratus regarded both *pneuma* and bodily heat as not innate but acquired from outside.[432] He distinguished between merely vital *pneuma*, which sustained life and had its seat in the left ventricle of the heart, and mental *pneuma* (πνεῦμα ψυχικόν) which had its seat in the brain though reaching it through the heart and arteries.[433] *Pneuma* from the outer air reached the heart's left ventricle directly from the lungs through the pulmonary vein, and was distributed from the heart through the ascending and descending aorta. When breathed in it had a certain density without which it would have hampered respiration and caused death.[434] As proof of this he took what we call the carbonic acid poisoning and asphyxia which he thought followed from breathing in the air of caves and freshly painted rooms.[435]

On the flow of *pneuma* in the heart and vascular system a few points may be added to those already given. He regarded the pulse as due to movement of *pneuma* in the arteries, set going by the heart's contractions.[436] In the heart the diastole came first, to draw in *pneuma*; but in the arteries the diastole followed the movement of *pneuma*, and was not in time with the diastole of the heart, but followed on its systole.[437] That is to say, he saw arterial diastole as resulting from waves of pressure. The *pneuma* sent out by the heart could not return to it, being excluded by the auricular valves, but must have been conceived to issue through the skin into the outer air.[438] In spite of all this connection between respiration and heartbeat as affecting *pneuma*, however, Erasistratus did not maintain an illusory correspondence in time between them.

In his account of the heart he distinguished the sigmoid or semilunar valves which blocked the return of *pneuma* from the aorta and the pulmonary artery, the tricuspid valves which stopped blood and *pneuma* from going out of the heart by the way they had entered, and the bicuspid valve of the pulmonary vein which had the same function.[439] While Herophilus had regarded the auricles as part of the heart, Erasistratus appears to have taken them as part of the great vessels.[440] He also discovered the chyle ducts of the intestines, but did not see their importance for renewing the blood. He regarded them as a special kind of artery containing first *pneuma* and later a milky humour.[441] He had a good knowledge of the main vessels nourishing the various parts of the trunk: the great *arteria* (our aorta) and descending aorta running in front of the spine, the intercostal *arteriae*, branches of the descending aorta reaching single ribs, the *arteriae* supplying the kidneys and the stomach, the 'smooth *arteria*' (our pulmonary vein), and among veins the *vena cava* rising from the left atrium near the aorta, the *vena azygos* running by the spine as far as the diaphragm and the intercostal veins branching from it, the artery-like vein, as Herophilus had called it, leading to the liver (our portal vein) and the hepatic veins that join the *vena cava*.[442] Yet theory still required him to say that only the veins in this list carried blood, the arteries being full of *pneuma*.

In the treatment of patients he distinguished, like his predecessors, between hygiene, the maintenance of health, including prevention of disease, and therapy, the treatment of disease once it had appeared.[443] Of these, he valued hygiene more. The expert on hygiene must pay close attention to his patient's habits of life; evacuations which seem to do little good must not be interrupted or the patient will become ill. In diagnosis Erasistratus thought that attention should be diverted from close examination of all symptoms to the discovery of the causes of the illness, even if they were remote; such remote causes he called *προκαταρκτικά* and *προηγούμενα αἴτια*, originating and antecedent, and thought them more important than those causes, more immediately observable, which the Empiric sect considered alone worthy of notice.[444] This opinion shows a scientist's confidence in a long chain of causes for presently observed phenomena, but must have differed in important details from the facile use of general causes that was a defect of pre-Socratic speculation.

Like the Hippocratics, Erasistratus insisted that treatment must vary according to individual needs. He rejected all violent methods, such as drastic purges, particularly in cases of inflamed joints and gout.[445] He did not ban all bleeding, unlike his master Chrysippus, but he limited it severely.[446] In haemorrhages he prescribed swaddling of the extremities, particularly of the shoulders and groin, with woollen bandages.[447] This was to counteract the lethally weakening effect of bleeding after the fasting which was part of the treatment for haemorrhage.[448] While the limbs were bandaged, bleeding was carried out from the breast, so that anastomosis of vessels could close and there would be enough nourishment to maintain life in the bandaged parts.[449] Morbid matters were also to be drawn off by vomiting, sweat, urine and hot baths. But most of the morbid excesses were to be prevented by diet, exercise, baths and even vomiting in the manner of the Hippocratic books on regimen. Massage, unguents and diuretics were favourite remedies of his. Cold baths were forbidden, particularly at the beginning of treatment.[450] His forms of regimen were no less costly than the Hippocratics'.

In surgery he could be bold. Empyema between the peritoneum and the intestines was removed by operation.[451] The abdomen was opened for applying remedies directly to the liver.[452] But he thought paracentesis superfluous and even dangerous treatment for dropsy, because the fluid always formed again, and because the diaphragm and the organs below it were drawn into sharing the disease when the fluid was drained off.[453] When there was abdominal paralysis he relieved stranguria with an S-shaped catheter invented by himself.[454] In pathology Erasistratus practised necropsy, demonstrating stony hardness of the liver, and palsy of the colon and bladder in snake-bite.[455]

Herophilus and Erasistratus thus made great progress in medical science and in therapy, so that medicine seemed destined for more triumphs in Alexandria. But after their generation we find little improvement. There may even have been a loss of skill in succeeding generations. The immediate cause was not, as yet, in any change of policy made by the Ptolemies, who had provided the background and the facilities that these scientists enjoyed. These included not only the privileges of the Museum, but widespread commercial contact with oriental countries, including India, from which drugs and remedies were imported. There appears to have been a change of tone among the Alexandrian physicians themselves, which weakened their impetus in discovery and diverted some of their intellectual energies to less profitable ends. The decline appears in medical knowledge and in surgery. It is hardly accurate to say that mere growth of specialisms was enough to bring it about even in surgery, for specialisms in the modern sense, concerned with particular organs, did not yet exist, though the Cnidian tradition sometimes pointed the way. The cause is rather that Alexandrian medicine became divided, in the manner of contemporary philosophy and later theology, into sects whose quarrels were more important to them than the advance of knowledge which might have been achieved by using the ideas of another sect.

In surgery, for instance, the main advances had been made by Erasistratus, with his new knowledge of anatomy. He had, as we saw, opened the flanks of patients in order to spread remedies directly on the liver, and had then sewn up the tissues again. In order to decide upon puncturing the abdomen to drain the fluid collected in the kind of dropsy called *ascites*, which made the patient bulge like a wineskin, he must have made inspections of this operation, and of its result, namely, that the fluid gathered again very quickly. He believed that dropsy was a disease of the liver to be cured by internal medicine.[456]

Celsus remarks that when surgery became a specialism in Alexandria it collected its experts from other branches of medicine.[457] Of these one of the most famous was Philoxenus, who wrote voluminous works and was an expert on cancer. Among those which earlier writers had called hidden he mentioned particularly cancers of the womb and of the intestines.[458] With Apollonius and Sostratus, he was insistent that a growth occupying the neck of the womb and the vagina must as far as possible be removed from the roots and the wound treated with equal care.[459] If this is cervical cancer in the developed state we may wonder how often the patient was cured. But the short accounts of these surgeons mention various kinds of tumours. This was a development beyond the Hippocratics. So was the technique attributed to Ammonius of crushing a stone in the incised bladder with a blunt-ended instrument pressed against a hooked one.[460]

The surgery of fractured and dislocated bones continued on ultimately Hippocratic lines but with considerable help from the ὀργανικοί, makers and users of surgical apparatus, who became a special profession during this period. These men depended for custom and patients on the surgeons proper. One of them was Apollonius the Mechanic, who has to be distinguished from the surgeons Apollonius the Mouse, Apollonius the Brute, and Apollonius the Snake, of various dates.[461] On these Alexandrian surgeons and their successors research is proceeding through scattered texts.[462] It appears that in Alexandria they became gradually separated from other practitioners (perhaps because they were less argumentative), until in later antiquity, and for long afterwards, professional surgery came to be regarded as an undignified craft, though physicians of standing might sometimes perform operations, as Galen did.

In a sense the decline of medicine in Alexandria may be said to have begun in the lifetime of Herophilus and Erasistratus, with the Empirics.[463] These were the first example of a medical sect, a new phenomenon that arose in Alexandria. The medical schools of earlier times, such as the Coan and the Cnidian, for whom no collective noun such as σχολή was usually employed, had begun as local groups of practitioners having traditions both of doctrine and of treatment. Within a general framework of common assumptions, their differences concerned fact and practice. The sects, or αἱρέσεις, on the other hand, took up doctrinaire attitudes, which owed much to the philosophers, to the whole of medicine. Practical treatment of many ailments might not differ much from one sect to another, but their differences in theoretical views of medical science were often extreme. Once more philosophy made its influence felt in medicine – indeed, scientific medicine during its career at Alexandria was never really independent of philosophy except in the humblest of practical activities. Unlike philosophy in our own day, which has increasingly parted company with science and with concrete knowledge, Greek philosophy was the most powerful force in the intellectual life of antiquity.[464]

Thus the differences between the sects lay in their philosophical approach and depended comparatively little on actual evidence in the settling of disputed points. The medical sects were indeed linked to philosophical sects. Thus the Empiric sect had its links with the Sceptics of the New Academy at Athens.[465] Its earliest figure, according to Galen, was Philinus, originally from Cos and a pupil of Herophilus.[466] His younger contemporary Serapion of Alexandria appears in Celsus as the founder and is also prominent in Galen.[467] The charge made by these two men against the medicine that they knew in Alexandria was that it had more and more abandoned the firm ground of experience and submitted itself to certain theoretical doctrines which had become fixed systems more respected than experience. This philosophical system-making in the field of medicine was the work of writers whom the Empirics called δογματικοί; the Dogmatists indeed counted as a sect in the later history of medicine.[468] The Empirics' rebellion against excessive use of the unaided intellect to form binding theories in medicine was stimulated by the example of Pyrrho and his Sceptic followers in the Academy, who rejected systematized Platonism.[469] The longest and the most important of extant accounts of Empiric doctrine is in the *Empiric Outline* (Ὑποτύπωσις ἐμπειρική) of Galen, which is preserved only in a Latin rendering entitled *Subfiguratio Empirica*.[470]

Like the Sceptics, the Empirics denied that there could be absolutely objective knowledge, which in medicine was systematic physiology, covering many things not directly accessible to the senses. They did not deny the senses in order to put their trust in something else, but based themselves exclusively on direct and sensible experience in the examination of patients. They held that enquiry about obscure causes and natural actions was superfluous because nature was not to be comprehended.[471] Like a farmer or a pilot, the physician was made by practice. It was practice, indeed, which produced the knowledge about which theoreticians argued.[472] They condemned vivisection as not only cruel but useless, because, when the body was laid open, even immediately after vivisection, the colour, smoothness, softness, hardness and such qualities of its parts would still not be the same as in the untouched body.[473] But they allowed some usefulness to anatomy.

Thus much of their argument recalls the attitude of the Hippocratic *Ancient Medicine*, but it is doctrinally reinforced. Celsus himself comments that Hippocrates, Erasistratus and others, who were not content to busy themselves over fevers and ulcerations but also searched out the nature of things, did not become just practitioners thereby, but became better practitioners.[474]

The Empirics from Serapion onwards formulated a theory of medical inference and procedure just as elaborately as if they had been philosophers of the Academy. For them the true source of human knowledge was observation (τήρησις); the Greek word implies careful and continual watching with the use of memory. This needed to be reinforced by historical tradition (ἱστορία), that is, records of other people's observations, since for well-grounded generalization one human life might not be long enough. Serapion added as a further resource analogical inference (μετάβασις τοῦ ὁμοίου). These three methods were called the 'tripod', the base with three legs.

For the fundamental activity of observation they naturally made rules.[475] The basis for organized and useful observation was in experience (πεῖρα, sometimes called αὐτοψία), which in their classification had two divisions: accidental or unpremeditated experience (αὐτοματική) and experiment (αὐτοσχέδιος), which however was far from being scientific experiment in the modern sense. An example is given of this kind of experiment: a traveller attacked and wounded by a wild beast and having none of the usual herbs with him might apply some other herb which he saw growing in the place, and this herb might have as good an effect as known remedies. Even prompting by a dream to use some substance might come under this head. In the first case there is no careful preparation but only improvisation to meet a need; especially there is no system of conditions set up to test a preconceived hypothesis, such as is necessary in modern sciences for useful experiment. But information obtained in this way was tested and watched in repetition (μιμητική πεῖρα). Like modern scientists the Empirics said that single cases were outside science, and that collections of instances were necessary before the general propositions of which science consists (θεωρήματα) could be made.[476] Thus the Empiric lore concerning observation and experiment shows beginnings of the approach elaborated in modern science. It also made full allowance for individual differences between patients, the more so because medical rules and procedures rest on the knowledge derived from concrete cases.

This might seem a very admirable and enlightened attitude to science, particularly to medical science. But the emphasis on the observable was overdone; it cramped the legitimate use of hypothesis and the imagination required for guessing the character of processes which were not directly accessible to observation, yet did have important consequences. Science, including medical science, has made much progress since by bringing unobservable things within the reach of observation, either directly by new techniques, or indirectly by forms of measurement very closely affected by things which still cannot be observed.

Thus in their view of disease the Empirics looked for every feature which was not natural to the body (παρὰ φύσιν), and called these individual symptoms. Diseases were complexes (συνδρομαί) of symptoms. Remedies were applied largely to single or isolable symptoms without any general theory of cause for the disease. The disease was an entity constructed for the time being by the intellect, and might indeed be repeated in many cases with its constituent symptoms, which were then called 'reminding signs' (ὑπομνηστικὰ σημεῖα).[477] Some symptoms were peculiar to individuals and some were repeated from case to case. This is all obvious enough, but the Empirics went so far in this phenomenalist and nominalist attitude as to reject all general causes, not only the discredited humours of tradition, but many others too. Thus the subject-matter of medicine became for them so multiple and so little ordered that medicine was no longer a science, and it became common in later ages to condemn those who treated superficial symptoms as 'mere Empirics'. Some conception of depth or generality of causes is a necessity of medical science. This need the Dogmatists on their side continually tried to meet, but much of their argument, as Galen pointed out, led from the visible to the invisible, so that conclusions could not be tested.

A great variety of subjects has been treated in this chapter. The developments which have been traced are all part of the complex history of Alexandrian science, which was affected by ideas from many parts of the Greek world and from beyond. This combination of wealth, power, and intellectual sophistication in one great city was peculiar to Alexandria, though there were other great cities in the Hellenistic world. Medicine was intensively studied in the Museum, and those who were trained there carried their learning and their attitudes elsewhere, particularly, in the next age, to Rome. For some time Alexandria remained the only centre where human anatomy could be learned directly by dissection, though that facility finally disappeared in the Roman period.

CHAPTER VII

MEDICINE FROM THE ALEXANDRIANS TO GALEN

THIS CHAPTER IS INTENDED to continue the story of Greek medicine from the Alexandrian decline to the moment before Galen attempted to make a synthesis of known medicine, at least in outline. Historically and socially the period is one of complex developments in the Hellenistic and Roman worlds. The impetus of Alexandrian discovery dies down, though here and there practical improvements continue. But physicians trained in Alexandria reach other parts of the Greek world or of the Roman empire, and Alexandrian doctrines continue to be spread. The bulk of written sources is again very great towards the end of the period, greater indeed than that of the Hippocratic Corpus even if Galen's own works alone are reckoned. But there is not space to treat or illustrate these sources fully, nor is this warranted by important novelties in their contents. Indeed, much time was taken up in Alexandrian and Roman times with comments on the Hippocratic writings, which by a sort of inertia gradually recovered their authority.

It seems best to give some shape and direction to this material by pursuing at first the history of the medical sects of the later kind, other than the Empirics already treated, namely the Dogmatists, Methodists and Pneumatists. All these are different from the Herophileans and Erasistrateans, who merely maintained the opinions of their original masters and founders without adding to knowledge. The Empirics and Dogmatists, as we saw, had their origins in Alexandria, like the Herophileans and Erasistrateans whom Galen also criticizes. But the Methodists and Pneumatists arose later and elsewhere. The sects survived their critic Galen – to whom we are indebted for most of our information about them – for a considerable time, and some had an influence which outlasted antiquity. But from the point of view of medieval medicine Galen appeared to have included, judged and superseded their teaching in his own system, as Aristotle considered himself to have done with the pre-Socratic philosophers.

A link between Alexandrian medicine and the medical sects of Roman times is the eminent physician Asclepiades of Bithynia, disciple of Erasistratus and believer in atomism, who had studied at least in Athens before he came to Rome.[478] During this earlier part of his life he was a professional rhetorician, even at Rome, where he was an elder contemporary of Lucretius. At Rome he changed course and became a physician; it appears that this had been his father's profession. Asclepiades rejected the humoral physiology and pathology as Erasistratus had done, incurring the censure of Galen for this rebellion against Hippocrates, a name which stood for traditional medicine even of the most ossified kind.

Much of Asclepiades' doctrine is likely to go back ultimately to the Peripatetics. In his general physiology he applied the atomic theory strictly. He accepted the difference between vital and mental *pneuma* and took the brain as the centre of the latter. The finest atoms were those of *pneuma* which were collected in the breast by inspiration before they reached the brain. The crowding or rarefaction of these atoms determined the state of the body, crowding being the cause of pain if not of disease.[479]

To show that the brain was the particular seat of *pneuma* Asclepiades carried out experiments illustrating the effects of decapitation on eels, tortoises, goats, crickets and flies. These creatures did survive for a while but in varying degrees.[480] Mental derangement he treated by physical means, using music and other influences to affect the brain.[481] He believed that the atoms of *pneuma* in the brain were rounded and smoother and thus more volatile than those of the rest of the body, which were held together by hooks.[482] In general theory he annoyed the Empirics by arguing that the isolated observations in which they trusted could never be repeated in identical conditions.

In treatment he denounced the excessive use of emetics and purges, but allowed that bleeding, clysters and cupping-glasses had their usefulness. Though he was the last Democritean atomist in medical theory, he did bequeath to the Methodists enough of this doctrine to be the base of their doctrine of close-packed and relaxed states of the body.[483]

The continual friction between Empiricists and Dogmatists is described by Galen in his essays *On Sects* and *On Medical Experience for New Entrants*.[484] It is a phase of the ceaseless argument in science between the champions of theory and of observation, both of which are necessary. In this argument the Empirics certainly scored points but they did not in the long run help the advance of medicine, since single phenomena, or even repeated phenomena of the same kind, do not make science until they are combined with others into a general structure. An attempt to steer a middle course between these attitudes was made by the Methodists, who are important in the history of medicine in spite of the fact that their doctrine as simply stated was jejune and absurd. They appear to have taken much of their attitude from Aenesidemus, a later Sceptic of the Academy, just as the Empirics did from earlier Sceptics.[485]

The Methodist tradition appears to have derived from Themison, a pupil of Asclepiades, though ancient authorities, such as Celsus, Soranus and Galen, do not make him the actual founder and even sometimes contrast him with the Methodists.[486] In fact there is no agreement on the founder. From Asclepiades Themison derived the theory of the body as made of small particles, whether Democritean atoms or not, having pores between them. The pores were always important in Methodist doctrine, since on their size and number depended the state of the body, dense, lax, or a mixture of the two. The crowding or rarefaction of these particles, already suggested by Asclepiades, was a favourite topic of Themison's.[487] In general acute diseases were due to crowding, *status strictus*, and chronic diseases due to rarefaction, *status laxus*, each state being more extreme than it should be. These universal states of the body (κοινότητες or *communitates*) were the foundation of Methodist lore. The general purpose of treatment was to dry or condense a body which was too soft or relaxed, and to relax a body which was too dense and dry. Between the two extremes they allowed a great variety of detail, especially when they were mixed so as to be different in different tissues. To this they added the effects of the environment, particularly of climate, and of poisons, tumours and the invasion of foreign bodies.[488] Treatment was suggested immediately, but apparently without exhaustive knowledge, by the state of the diseased place. In practice it consisted of the same baths, regimen and other remedies as were common in other kinds of medicine, though it was claimed that this was the result of true insight and not merely of observation on the spot, as with the Empirics. Not unnaturally Galen thought this 'method', or compromise between the Empiric and the Dogmatist views, a thing of little worth on its own account.[489] But at least one notable physician, Soranus, was trained in the school.

Somewhere in the Methodist succession the fixed doctrine of chronic and acute diseases was formulated. This dominated later medicine for centuries. Its most active propagator was Thessalus of Tralles, who attracted the attention of Nero, and incidentally claimed to be able to train a physician in six months.[490] His claim cannot have increased the reputation of the school among the thoughtful, though he did call himself ἰατρονίκης, 'the victor over physicians'. He was regarded as a figure of some importance even in Methodist doctrine, though he was not the founder of the sect. He did, however, attempt to strengthen its foundations and to extend and refine practice. From Aenesidemus the Methodists drew the philosophical principle that scientific knowledge of things unseen (ἄδηλα) was not so much impossible as useless. Thessalus defined medicine as the knowledge of the manifest universal qualities (again the κοινότητες or *communitates*) as relevant and necessary to health. The universal qualities, if out of balance, automatically compelled the physician to act.[491] This compulsion of sickness was the strongest element in Thessalus' doctrine. Beside it, any other kind of exact formulation or description counted for nothing; his medical language therefore reduced to indifferent synonyms the three usually distinct terms πάθος, νόσημα and σύμπτωμα. Crude heating or cooling, moistening or drying of the patient was fundamental.

Physiology, anatomy and even prognosis counted for nothing with him, nor even any systematic rules of hygiene. Thessalus also practised surgery. In therapy he attempted, on Themison's principles but without theoretical interest, to alter the composition or texture of the body. Whether he was treating a chronic condition or an ulcer he used means differing only according to the stage of the illness, beginning, increase, culmination or aftermath, which he thought he could forecast in a sequence of days.[492] This crude, brisk and confident manner of treatment had something in it which appealed to Romans, and was thought particularly useful for the ailments of slaves. The Methodist attitude, in his case more than others, recalls modern pragmatism, which has claimed to be a consciously healthy philosophy in a rough world. It may well have had its psychological advantages.

But the greatest figure in the Methodist sect, and indeed one of the greater physicians of antiquity considered in his own right, was Soranus, who is known chiefly as an obstetrician and gynaecologist, and as an authority on the treatment of infants, though the titles of his works on other subjects are known.[493] It is difficult to see how Methodist doctrine determined his opinions or limited his interests.

His work on gynaecology is preserved in a curious form. First there is a Latin translation by a certain Muscio of a work containing questions to be addressed to midwives and the correct answers, in two books.[494] Secondly there are Greek fragments of a longer work on gynaecology written in four books, which can be supplemented by passages translated into Latin by Caelius Aurelianus in his *Acute Diseases* and *Chronic Diseases*, datable perhaps to the fifth century.[495] Caelius Aurelianus was himself a Methodist, which shows the long endurance of the sect. Both the books of questions and answers and the larger *Gynaecology* (*Περὶ γυναικείων*) are very practical and have been admired in later ages, though Soranus was not a specialist in gynaecology in the modern sense.

The *Midwives' Catechism* (*Περὶ τῆς γενησομένης μαίας*) was a sort of elementary extract from the larger *Gynaecology*. The first two books of the *Gynaecology* deal with those who are to become midwives, with those who have become midwives, with duties that fall to the midwife in health or in sickness, with the anatomy of the female organs, with menstruation, conception, pregnancy and the care of pregnant women, and with their *picas* or cravings. The first book touches on the growth of the embryo, the means for easy delivery, difficult delivery, miscarriage and abortion; abortion is not to be carried out when precipitated by adultery or in order to preserve beauty, but only for strictly medical reasons such as the insufficient size of the organs, neoplasms or lesions. But a long list of contraceptive methods is given, with a warning against those that are too drastic. The second book deals with the signs that birth is near and with the care necessary at this stage, with preparations for birth and birth itself, procedure for bringing out a retained afterbirth, and the care of the new mother and her baby. The midwife has to declare the sex of the baby and convince herself that it is worth rearing – surely a heavy responsibility. Directions are given for cutting the navel string with a surprising variety of instruments from nails and shells to surgical instruments of iron. The first washing and the swaddling of the baby, its bed and its feeding follow. There is no strict demand that the mother should suckle it in all circumstances. When there is a danger of the mother's premature ageing or wasting her place must be taken by a wet-nurse.

Both midwife and wet-nurse must be chosen carefully. The midwife must have the right mental, moral and physical qualities; she must be literate and study her work theoretically. She must have a keen understanding and a good memory, must enjoy her work and have a sense of honour, must have sound sense, a strong constitution, practical experience and presence of mind, must not be easily alarmed, but must be sympathetic; that she should herself have given birth is not absolutely necessary. She should further be strong, steady, not given to talk, proof against bribery by those who desire criminal abortion and free of superstition. Finally she must have gentle hands. These good qualities must have been hard to find in one woman, except for families of means, such as Soranus' patients probably were.

The wet-nurse should not be younger than twenty or older than forty. She must already have borne two or three children, be healthy, strong, plump and blooming; her breasts should be normal, relaxed, soft and unwrinkled, the nipples neither too large nor too small, too hard nor too spongy; she must be even-tempered, charming, gentle, a Greek and clean. Her milk must be of just the right kind and her manner of life and regimen strictly controlled. When the mother's milk is inadequate in quantity and quality the wet-nurse should take over, but measures should be taken to restore the mother. The perfect wet-nurse too must have been hard to find, if these were her qualities.

Among details of feeding the child, the first solid food is recommended to be given at six months, but weaning will not be complete until eighteen months or two years have passed. When a child is very thirsty after food, water or watery wine should be given through artificial teats. Unfortunately Soranus does not mention the material of which these teats were made; what can it have been in a world which did not yet use rubber? Nor does he mention any such vessels as our babies' bottles, to which they might have been attached. The great length of time before weaning is still found among peoples who have not an adequate milk supply.

Infants' diseases or disorders are treated next: inflamed tonsils, rashes, itches, catarrh, coughs, touches of sun, feverish conditions affecting the brain and diarrhoea.

The two later books deal with the diseases of women as contrasted with men, with conditions which are contrary to nature (*παρὰ φύσιν*). Dietetic healing is recommended for menstrual troubles, and for various conditions of the uterus such as swellings, hardenings, moles and bleeding, displacement and even sterility. Medicine, gymnastic exercises and psychological treatment are mentioned, including such things as protective amulets, approved for their suggestive effect. But he condemns fumigation of the uterus as likely to produce only ulcers; also flashing lights and the beating of cauldrons and kettle-drums whose noise alone would give a healthy woman a headache. The last two remedies must surely have belonged to magic, and have been intended to drive out or repel demons.

The fourth book treats of afflictions remedied by surgery and drugs: abscesses, tumours, cancers, fistulae, haemorrhoids and the like. A Methodist feature of his doctrine here is that surgery should not be used unless the universal conditions cannot be remedied by medicine, applied or taken internally.

Soranus illustrated his larger *Gynaecology* and probably also the *Catechism*. The illustrations show the form of the uterus and its parts, and the position of the foetus *in utero*, and are preserved in many manuscripts. The information given and the treatment recommended must belong to a tradition of great antiquity, grounded in folk medicine, illuminated by the rational medicine of the Hippocratics and Alexandrians, and no doubt improved in technical details and in equipment during the Roman period.

On the physiology of reproduction in general Soranus also wrote a book entitled *Semen and the Generation of Animals* (*Περὶ σπέρματος καὶ ζωογονίας*).[496] He wrote another on pathology, *Acute and Chronic Diseases* (*Περὶ ὀξέων καὶ χρονίων παθῶν*), and various works on pharmacology, ophthalmology, general surgery, bandaging and poisons, all of these surviving only in fragments or allusions.[497] His gynaecological work must have survived because of its practical value.

Last among the medical sects to be considered are the Pneumatists. They too have their philosophical affiliation, which was chiefly to the Stoics, as will be shown, though they appear to have had links with the Peripatetic tradition of science. Their doctrine had a long ancestry, since it goes back to the general tradition of *pneuma* as vital air which is so prominent in some of the Hippocratic books, such as *The Sacred Disease*, and, in its different fashion, *Breaths*, and was still an influence on Diocles and Praxagoras. The compiler of *Anonymus Londinensis*, in its final form, also appears to have been a Pneumatist. It was natural that *pneuma* should continue as one of the important conceptions of Greek medicine; it survived in later medicine too, and as we saw earlier the problems which it was intended to solve were not put into proper form until the discovery of oxygen and of its part in biochemistry.[498]

The founder of Pneumatism was Athenaeus of Attalia in Pamphylia, who was a pupil of the well-known Stoic philosopher and scientist Posidonius of Apamea.[499] The sect was founded about the middle of the first century BC and not later, as some scholars used to maintain. It is not mentioned by Celsus, but that is not conclusive evidence for a later date. By the first century AD, on the other hand, most of the established Pneumatist physicians are likely to have had contact with Rome, if not to have lived there. The only Pneumatist whose work is preserved in its entirety is Aretaeus, who belongs to this century.[500] But the best physician of the school appears to have been Archigenes, who enquired carefully into the original seats of diseases which subsequently affected other parts and into sympathetic pains, and distinguished primary from secondary symptoms. He was also an admired surgeon.[501]

The Pneumatists were not all strict followers of the doctrine, for some left the fold with Agathinus of Sparta, founder of the Eclectics, who combined Pneumatist doctrines with others, and committed themselves entirely to no school or sect.[502] The Eclectics themselves are sometimes reckoned a sect, but their attitude really precludes this title. Some were rather Sceptics than Stoics in philosophy and more like the Empirics in their medical views. Their other title, Episynthetics, indicated that they put together the opinions of others by way of afterthought. Their line of tradition was later represented by the surgeon Leonidas of Alexandria and the physician Archigenes of Apamea. They were in full vigour in the time of Galen.

In the tradition ancestral to Pneumatism one innovation appears to have been made in the Peripatetic essay *On Spirit* (*Περὶ πνεύματος*), where it is said that *pneuma* is not the whole of soul but contributes to the potentiality of it.[503] It has been argued that this author believed in a separate soul-stuff which was not one of the four elements, but a fifth. But the Pneumatist doctrine of later times took *pneuma* as a compound in varying proportions of air and fire. For the Stoics *pneuma* pervaded the universe and was the vehicle of cosmic *sympatheia*, the power by which every part of the universe was sensitive to events in every other part. It bore some resemblance to the physical field which in modern physics has superseded the solid physical object having only one or only a simple location. According to the Stoic theory of tension (*τόνος*) movements were propagated immediately out to the edge and then back to the centre of the universe, and on the microcosmic scale likewise within any smaller object.

This Stoic doctrine has been compared to the modern conception in physics of the propagation of a state without the transport of matter, as found in the wave motion of ripples in water, or of sound in the air, both of them naturally known and discussed by the Stoics, or less obviously in the physical fields of radiation, electricity and magnetism.[504] It was always sharply opposed to the Democritean atomism adopted by the Epicurean philosophers, and, as we saw, by some Alexandrian thinkers in medicine. Within medicine Pneumatists did not need to think in terms of agglomerations of atoms, transient or lasting, and of pores between them, as Asclepiades and the Methodists did. On the contrary, using this cosmic model with its property of tension or the propagation of states, they were able to conceive of the *pneuma* in the nerves as communicating states from the seat of intelligence outwards to the surface and back again. For the Stoics, even for Posidonius, the centre of intelligence continued to be the heart, as with the Sicilian physicians and with Aristotle. This last doctrine, while it was still accepted in medicine, must have made difficulties for Pneumatists, who were acquainted with the Alexandrian discovery of nerves, but they seem to have insisted on restoring the heart as the centre of consciousness.

The general theory of tension in a field which included the centre, wherever it might be placed, and its radiating nerves or vessels was much nearer to our own view of nervous action than early notions of the flow of air or *pneuma* from one part to another (as in *The Sacred Disease*, for all that book's recognition of the brain).

The Pneumatists under Stoic influence were thus largely regressive in their physiology, in spite of some insights. They took a more rational view of malformation of the genitals than some physicians, and were prepared to operate on the male organs. They made great use of baths in their treatment. But their view of disease as a fixed entity without process was not useful to medicine.

Such were the sects of later Greek medicine, each having characteristic defects due largely to the strongly philosophical framework in which they grew up. But the philosophy of their own age or of slightly earlier periods gave direction and shape to their thought. It was not necessarily a disadvantage that the philosophical doctrines should be consciously held, for in our own time there is too much unexamined assumption in some scientific work and even thought. The still undivorced state of philosophy and science, an inheritance from the Ionian nature philosophers, was not necessarily an evil, in spite of some bizarre opinions which permeated early thought on science.

During the same period another important figure, Rufus of Ephesus, remains to be treated.[505] He was born under Trajan, spent much time in Egypt and may have lived for a time at Rome. He is mentioned with respect by Galen, and like him belonged to no sect.[506] The style of his written remains is lucid and sensible, and his thought clear. He was both practitioner and theoretician, well acquainted with Aristotle as well as with the Hippocratic writings. He compared the anatomy of men and apes, and discovered the decussation of the optic nerve fibres on the ventral surface of the brain, as well as blood-vessels in the uterus which had previously not been known. He seems to have contributed to the diagnosis of the pulse, later to be a favourite study of Galen's. He also distinguished himself in medical botany, on which he wrote four books in hexameters, reviving a habit of the Alexandrians.

His writings, though not so numerous as Galen's, appear to have covered general anatomy and anatomical nomenclature, regimen, the condition of the blood, the theory of the pulse, diseases of the kidneys and bladder, satyriasis and gonorrhoea, diseases of the joints, acute and chronic diseases, fevers, gynaecology and obstetrics, external ulcers and tumours, diseases of the eye, studies of urine, and a variety of pharmacological topics, on which he was expert. He also wrote on melancholia and hydrophobia. Like others, he commented on Hippocrates.

The physicians mentioned here were the near-predecessors or contemporaries of Galen, to whom we are indebted for much of our information about them. We come next to Galen himself.

CHAPTER VIII

GALEN

THE PROPER TREATMENT OF GALEN is something of a problem in a short survey such as this. Should his works be treated as a new and extensive territory in their own right, or should they form a boundary-stone to end our account?

The second of these treatments is required by limitations of space and can also be excused by the bulk and nature of his surviving writings, which, though they are the work of one man, extend by themselves to twice the length of the Hippocratic Corpus.[507] A large part of them consists of commentaries on well-known Hippocratic books, commentaries which are usually much longer than those books themselves. Some again are intended for readers whom we should today call medical students, since their titles contain the phrase *τοῖς εἰσαγομένοις*, 'for recruits to the profession'. Some of the longest are like our medical textbooks, whose authors' business is to set forth the existing state of knowledge and practice in particular fields, and not to present the results of new researches of their own. Galen's medical textbooks of this kind cannot readily be compared with the work of his predecessors, which has mostly perished apart from his own summaries and criticisms. His own contributions to medical science are not always easy to determine. But his general view of medicine and his ordering of its branches have a special importance for their effect on the later history of medicine. So too have his ethical and philosophical views. For he was highly educated in philosophy and took a technical interest in logical questions which has been a great benefit to modern historians of logic.

His own life also gives valuable evidence for the history of medicine as a career in ancient times, though some of it belongs to the history of Roman rather than of Greek medicine.[508] He was the son of an architect, Nicon of Pergamum, and in his youth attended the philosophical schools, where he became an expert in Aristotle's writings. Later he studied anatomy at Smyrna, and finally at Alexandria he completed his training with dissections. Returning to Pergamum, he became surgeon to a school of gladiators, where he gained much valuable experience. He arrived at Rome in 162, preceded by his fame, but in 166 left Italy for home, to avoid an outbreak of plague. Recalled by Marcus Aurelius in 169 to be his personal physician, he continued in this post until later that year Marcus asked him to accompany him on campaign on the Danube. He persuaded Marcus to release him from this duty on condition that he attended Commodus, heir to the throne. His motive was that he wished to continue his writing and scientific work, such as animal vivisection, while acting as physician at the imperial court in Rome. He died in 201, it is uncertain where. He thus enjoyed every advantage for pursuing his profession, including the leisure to write his numerous works.

He himself divided these into seven groups: anatomy, pathology, therapy, diagnostic and prognostic, commentaries on Hippocrates, philosophy and grammar. Among the medical works as thus classified there is no separate heading for physiology, but if we make this heading we may include under it such books as *On the Natural Faculties* (*Περὶ φυσικῶν δυνάμεων*), *On the Use of the Parts of the Human Body* (*Περὶ χρείας μορίων*) and his works on respiration, on the pulse, on embryology, and on the special sense organs.[509] The total number of Greek texts is more than one hundred and thirty in Kühn's edition, and there are some works preserved in Arabic translation only.[510] Some of the texts preserved under his name are spurious, as might be expected.[511] Only the most general account of his thinking can be presented here.

His system of medicine was pervaded by philosophical ideas, as were those of the sects mentioned in the last chapter. The ideas were mainly Aristotelian, but some of his attitudes were Platonic, and he had a tincture of Stoicism. Some of his works, which treat of logic and ethics, are not directly relevant to an account of his medicine. But he did set forth his philosophical attitude in one short tract, *That the Best Physician is Also a Philosopher* (ὅτι ὁ ἄριστος ἰατρὸς καὶ φιλόσοφος) – an opinion that was contrary to the doctrine and practice of such men as the Empirics.[512] Galen wished to revive the programme of the Hippocratic *Airs, Waters, Places* in studying the effects of the physical environment on health: to know the nature and texture of all parts of the body so as to determine their functions and interrelation and understand their diseases. Such theoretical studies, which he regarded as demonstrable knowledge, were needed for a good physician. In this sketch a deductive cast of mind appears, claiming too much for mere ratiocination.

In another, *On Medical Experience* (Περὶ τῆς ἰατρικῆς ἐμπειρίας), almost all of which is preserved for us only in an Arabic version, a long debate is presented between Dogmatists and Empirics; no conclusive judgment is made by Galen in favour of one side or the other, though the course of the argument favours the Empirics.[513] The Dogmatists put all their faith in the *logos*, which is equivalent to our term 'theory'. It alone singles out causes and relevant considerations, neglecting a mass of attendant circumstances. The Empiric requirement of seeing a phenomenon many times before judging is ridiculed because the required number of times cannot be stated, while one penetrating observation and judgment according to the *logos* is sufficient. Sophistical puzzles such as 'How many grains make a heap? How great a height makes a mountain? How many sheep make a flock?' are also mentioned in the Dogmatists' armoury, but are not accepted by Galen as being really relevant to the useful accumulation of observations. We can see that they require a false precision and certainty; the questions that they raise as applied to medical observation would now be regarded as statistical. Of similar interest is the passage where ἀναλογισμός, argument from the seen to the unseen which does not return to phenomena, is dismissed in favour of ἐπιλογισμός, argument from the seen back again to the seen.[514] The problems arising here, if they are pressed, will turn out to be those of inductive reasoning on connections. In spite of his Platonic training Galen is forced by his profession to be more empirical.

But he still maintained the Aristotelian teleology, the doctrine of the purposiveness of the body and its component parts. As a philosopher, indeed, in the *Use of Parts*, he even attributed the adaptations made by nature to God as *demiurgos*, using the word applied by Plato to the executant creator in the *Timaeus* but really meaning not a personal creator but an immanent reason or *logos* as conceived by the Stoics.[515] The Aristotelian doctrine of *entelecheia*, of the development of things to what they are normally destined to become, as the acorn to become the oak, was part of his thought. This adaptation of an organ to its function was a normal concept of biology and medicine in antiquity, as now. The adaptation is a supreme example of *techne*, as nature practises it. But Galen did not assume a craftsman standing outside nature, in spite of some of his language about the absolute goodness of the cosmos. Like Aristotle's, his was an immanent teleology not a theory of divine intervention.

In physiology Galen returned entirely to the humoral theory of the Hippocratics, as he also did for the foundations of his pathology. He wrote a whole treatise of his own with the title, *That the Character of the Soul Follows the Blending in the Body* (ὅτι ταῖς τοῦ σώματος κράσεσιν αἱ τῆς ψυχῆς δυνάμεις ἕπονται), that is, the blending of humours.[516] Once again, we are reminded by humoral theory of the modern accounts of endocrine secretions and their mental and emotional effects, the great difference being between the large quantities of the ancient humours and the small but powerful discharges of the ductless glands as we now know them. His theory of temperaments was a very important part of his physiology. After writing *The Elements according to Hippocrates* (Περὶ τῶν καθ' Ἱπποκράτην στοιχείων βιβλίον), he set out his own opinions in *Temperaments* (Περὶ κράσεων βιβλίον), in which he pursued the manifold combination of the four primary stuffs in healthy and in diseased bodies.[517] Each part of the body had its own blend (κρᾶσις) of these. The quality and nature of the whole body likewise varied with their interactions. In this line of thought is the origin of our word 'idiosyncrasy'; ἰδιοσυγκρασία does indeed occur once or twice in Galen's text.

Another book dealing with the material basis and the powers of the body is *On the Natural Faculties*, one of the best-known of

Galen's works and full of polemic against Chrysippus the Stoic and against Erasistratus.[518] Galen was as ready to reprove the great writers of the past as to quarrel with his contemporaries. The notion of δύναμις in this book is very pervasive and mostly verbal, being a development in medicine, not of δύναμις as known in *Ancient Medicine*, but of the Aristotelian δύναμις as potentiality contrasted with ἐνεργεία, activity or actuality, also Aristotelian. The faculties or powers of the body are primarily three, those of generation (compounded of alteration and shaping), of growth and of nutrition, and they have subordinated to them many specific and local faculties, as for instance blood-making, digestion and pulse. The full list recalls the conversation of Molière's physicians in *Le Malade Imaginaire*. Galen did do valuable work in dissection, however, correcting some of the results reached by earlier generations, and in the vivisection of animals for the furthering of neurology. He also proved that arteries as well as veins carry blood, a discovery that stands as a landmark in the history of Greek medicine.

In anatomy his most notable work is *Anatomical Procedures* (Ἀνατομικαὶ ἐγχειρήσεις), a medical textbook once more.[519] Book I describes the muscles and ligaments of the hand, Book II those of the legs, Book III the nerves and vessels of the limbs, Book IV the muscles of the head and neck, Book V the breast, the back and the belly. Book VI covers the alimentary tract, Books VII and VIII the respiratory organs, Book IX the brain and spinal marrow, Book X the eyes, tongue and oesophagus, Book XI the vascular system, Books XII and XIII the nervous system. This list includes nothing on the reproductive organs, male and female, perhaps because the outline given is otherwise common to both sexes. But Galen's other books do include one on the womb.[520] Closely connected with the strictly anatomical books are the works *On the Causes of Respiration* (Περὶ τῶν τῆς ἀναπνοῆς αἰτίων) and *On the Movement of Muscles* (Περὶ μυῶν κίνησεως).[521] His concern with the pulse is shown in the books *On the Use of Pulses* (Περὶ χρείας σφυγμῶν), *On Tremor, Palpitation, Convulsion and Rigor* (Περὶ τρόμου καὶ παλμοῦ καὶ σπασμοῦ καὶ ῥίγους βιβλίον), *On Pulses for Beginners* (Περὶ τῶν σφυγμῶν τοῖς εἰσαγομένοις), *On the Differences Between Pulses* (Περὶ *διαφορᾶς σφυγμῶν*), *On Distinguishing Pulses* (*Περὶ διαγνώσεως σφυγμῶν*), *On the Causes of Pulses* (*Περὶ τῶν ἐν τοίς σφυγμοῖς αἰτίων βιβλία*), *On Prognosis by Pulses* (*Περὶ προγνώσεως σφυγμῶν*) and *Synopsis of Pulses* (*Σύνοψις περὶ σφυγμῶν ἰδίας πραγματείας*).[522]

On regimen the most interesting books are *Theory of Health* (*Ὑγιεινῶν λόγος*), *On the Effects of Foods* (*Περὶ τροφῶν δυνάμεως*), *On Beneficial and Harmful Humours in Food* (*Περὶ εὐχυμίας καὶ κακοχυμίας τροφῶν*).[523]

In pathology Galen tried to combine two approaches which had little in common: the humoral, which he inherited from the Hippocratics, and the topographical and morphological, which originated with the Alexandrians. The defects of the humoral pathology, as of the corresponding physiology, must have been generally known in his time, but traditional piety, directed towards the figure called Hippocrates, was strong in Galen. Thus he still chose to classify diseases as due to yellow bile, black bile or phlegm, which could pervade the whole body or could strike particular organs.[524]

Among diseases or morbid conditions due to yellow bile, of which he distinguished seven types, were erysipelas, miliaria, herpes and other inflammations of the skin, which took on a straw-coloured appearance.[525] Jaundice of course is included, which is correct, but so are an inflammatory swelling which he calls elephantiasis, and *hydrops* (dropsy). The types of this bile were yellow (*ξανθή*), also called elementary bile, pale yellow (*ὠχρά*), reddish (*ἐρυθρά*), leek-green (*πρασώδης*), yolk-coloured (*λεκιθώδης*), rust-coloured (*ἰώδης*), and bluish or woad-coloured (*ἰσατώδης*). These colours in vomit or in excrement we have already seen in the clinical material from the Hippocratics. It has been remarked that bilirubin, the residue of red corpuscles that turns to bile, changes colour easily from yellow to green or reddish.[526] Thus there were definite phenomena to which this doctrine could be applied. Cirrhosis of the liver and haemolytic jaundice due to snake-bites were also thus explained.[527]

Black bile is, as we saw, a peculiar conception of ancient medicine which can be compared to no entity known in the modern science, least of all as a constituent of the body's fluids.[528] It was regarded as the cause of quartan fevers, leprosy and sometimes jaundice, and of many intestinal diseases, but most notably of the mental affliction called melancholia. Galen thought that he could detect it in the blood as a heavy sediment like the lees in wine. To it he himself attributed glandular diseases, including what we call Addison's disease, which is due to the failure of the adrenal glands and leaves dark pigment in the skin and mucous membranes. Galen called this 'black jaundice', comparing its colour to that of the black olive. He also detected black bile in the blood when the spleen failed to purge it. He was not certain whether the enlargement and hardening of the spleen which he saw in some fevers was also a toxic effect of black bile, but in this condition the spleen would absorb no more, and the bile was left to discolour the body and blood, causing low spirits and mental disturbance. He knew that this cirrhosis of the spleen was connected with cirrhosis of the liver. Other fevers, putrefaction, anthrax, carbuncle and even some cancers also appear in Galen as effects of black bile; and naturally also dysentery and cholera. Elephantiasis and leprosy are also added.

Phlegm, too, could cause various diseases.[529] It could, for instance, make a person more susceptible to quotidian fever. Fever in general arose when phlegm made the flesh swell up, or when phlegm and bile were retained in the same place and not cooled, and when nothing is excreted. Naturally the respiratory diseases, pneumonia, pleurisy and heavy catarrh, were attributed to phlegm. More surprising is the tracing of urinary stones to phlegm accumulated in the cavities of the kidneys and there consolidating. Watery phlegm in excess could cause dropsy in the forms called *tympanitis* and *ascites*, which distended the abdomen, and *anasarka*, which water-logged the whole body. Rheumatic heart disease and angina pectoris were also explained by phlegm.

Blood as the fourth humour could be excessive in quantity, the condition called plethora, or deficient, that is, in anaemia.[530]

From the Stoics Galen is likely to have got the germ of his doctrine of nerve-conduction and shock without transfer of matter. But he also believed in the spread of irritation by transfer of humours from one part to another.

His continuing belief in the humours prevented him from

gaining even more advantage than he did from the local pathology of his book *On Affected Places* (Περὶ τῶν πεπονθότων τόπων), where the organs are discussed in order with the signs and symptoms of their respective illnesses.[531] He lacked the knowledge which the best Alexandrians had had of morbid anatomy.

His greatest work on therapy was the long book *On the Method of Healing* (Μέθοδος θεραπευτική), intended to be a medical encyclopaedia covering the whole field for the benefit of practitioners.[532] There are fourteen books. Books I and II contain a violent polemic against the Methodist Thessalus, and lay the foundation for scientific method in healing; Books III–VI give general directions for treating lesions in particular organs, especially ulcers; Book VII, for treatment designed to restore a disturbed balance of humours as a cure for illness; Books VIII–XII give directions for the treatment of various kinds of fever, these too being signs of faulty mingling of elements in the entire body. Books XIII and XIV deal with tumours. Smaller writings were the earlier essay on *Unnatural Swellings* (Περὶ τῶν παρὰ φύσιν ὄγκων) and *Therapeutics* (Τῶν πρὸς Γλαυκῶνα θεραπευτικῶν βιβλίον) in two books.[533] A lost treatise in three books dealt with phlebotomy; but some idea of it can be gained from two small controversial essays, *On Phlebotomy Against Erasistratus* (Περὶ φλεβοτομίας πρὸς Ἐρασίστρατον) and *On Phlebotomy Against the Erasistrateans at Rome* (Περὶ φλεβοτομίας πρὸς τοὺς ἐν Ῥώμῃ Ἐρασιστρατείους), and also from a rather larger work, *A Therapeutic Treatise on Phlebotomy*[534] (Περὶ φλεβοτομίας θεραπευτικόν). Blood-letting was a practice based on theories of corrupted blood and of unbalanced humours. Erasistratus, as we saw, had no use for humoral theory.

Pharmacology was treated in three large treatises, *On the Mixing and Efficacy of Simple Drugs* (Περὶ τῶν ἁπλῶν φαρμάκων κρασέως καὶ δυνάμεως), in eleven books, *On the Compounding of Drugs for Local Application* (Περί συνθέσεως φαρμάκων τῶν κατὰ τόπους), in ten books, and *On the Compounding of Drugs According to their Kinds*[535] (Περὶ συνθέσεως φαρμάκων κατὰ γένη).

On surgery of the living body Galen wrote no separate treatise, though he did comment on the Hippocratic *Fractures* and *Joints*.[536] This was partly due to his standing preference for internal medicine wherever it could be used, but also to the demands of his system of medicine, dominated by the revived theory of humours, in which surgery could only be a little esteemed part of therapy. Another reason must have been the continually declining esteem of surgery in medical practice at large, which has been noted in Chapter 6 for the later Alexandrian and subsequent periods.

This attitude of Galen's was not altered by his experience at Pergamum as physician to the gladiators. Ordinary surgery of wounds, ulcers, tumours and other superficial damage or defects was also part of normal medicine, requiring no special training. On the Hippocratic treatment of broken bones Galen makes no comment which shows that any change had been made from the old practice in amputation. The Hippocratics did not make their cut nearly high enough in the sound flesh, but the Alexandrians came nearer to modern standards. Galen seems also to have been much more sparing than Hellenistic surgeons had been in the use of ligatures on blood-vessels to check bleeding.[537]

His eager interest in anatomy was diverted from practical use by his bitter controversies with the Erasistrateans of his own time and again limited by the framework of his general system. He mentions surgery from time to time, but very rarely surgeons, no doubt because they would need too prominent a place in his system. Surgery for him was apparently a form of aesthetic pruning of swellings, blemishes and such abnormalities as additional fingers beyond the usual five.[538] Thus the natural state would be restored and mutilation avoided.

He allowed exceptions to this general rule in some serious cases: in cutting for the stone, in removing cataract from the eye, in removing cancers absolutely when they were caught in a sufficiently early stage, and of course in obstetrics. But serious operations were only a last resort.[539] This was indeed a change from the practices of the great Alexandrians, and even from those of Praxagoras and Diocles, but it is hard to condemn Galen in his age and circumstances for lack of surgical boldness in his recommendations. It is exceedingly doubtful whether he himself practised any but superficial surgery. He actually says in one passage of his commentary on the Hippocratic *Joints* that he has omitted any account of later methods of extension and reduction because the subject is fully treated in the writings of the younger *organikoi*.[540]

Such is a brief notice of Galen's achievement in medicine. His philosophical preconceptions, persisting from his earlier education and maintained in the studies of his leisure, turned him eventually into a medical theologian, for whom anatomy was a form of praise and veneration of God. Like Plato and the Stoics, he was a firm monotheist, and as such he was acceptable alike to the Byzantine Christians, to the Latin Christians of Western Europe and to the Moslems, who took an intense interest in Greek science. He established an orthodoxy in medicine which he claimed to be above all the sects described in his writings. This might appear as a definite break with Greek medicine, but, as we saw, the philosophy contemporary with each age of medicine powerfully determined the physicians' cast of mind. The earliest Ionian nature philosophy was a form of theology, no less than the Platonism and Stoicism of later times.[541] In view of this history, it is not a matter for surprise that Galen ended as he did; it would rather have been surprising if he had taken any other course as the philosophical organizer of medical doctrine for his own time and for later ages.

CHAPTER IX

THE MEDICAL CAREER

THIS BOOK HAS BEEN CONCERNED with the general nature of Greek medicine as a tradition of practice and theory, and not more than incidentally with the medical career from the practitioner's point of view. Something indeed has been revealed by the Hippocratic Oath and the later writings on medical ethics and behaviour, but more needs to be said of the practitioner's life and circumstances as they may be reconstructed from our evidence.

Such evidence is not abundant before the middle of the fifth century, whatever may be inferred from the stories of mythical or legendary healers, or from the very general sketch of the physician's role given in *Ancient Medicine*. Even the lives and practice of Alcmaeon and Empedocles as physicians are very little known.

The first individual of note whose life story is told is Democedes of Croton, briefly mentioned in Chapter 2. He was clearly the product of a long tradition, that of the Western school with its Cnidian links. Most of our information about him comes from the well-known account in Herodotus already cited, to which the entry in the *Suda* under Δημοκήδης adds a little; something more may be gleaned from Athenaeus, Aelian and Iamblichus.[542] The full story may now be given to illustrate the rewards and the risks brought by medical skill. Democedes was the son of Calliphon, who had been priest of Asclepius at Cnidus before he moved his home to Croton. To escape his father's bad temper Democedes left for Aegina, where he practised without equipment until invited to become personal physician to Polycrates, tyrant of Samos, at a salary of two talents of gold. When

Polycrates was caught and killed by Oroetes, the satrap of Sardis, Democedes became the slave of Oroetes and remained in obscurity, not revealing his skill in medicine. Then, when Oroetes in his turn was put to death by order of Darius the Great King, Democedes' fortunes suddenly changed.

One day when he was out hunting Darius fell from his horse and dislocated his ankle very badly. The best of the Egyptian physicians at court used wrenching, which did not restore the bone but made the injury far worse, so that Darius could not sleep for seven days and nights. Then it was reported to Darius that among the slaves brought from the household of Oroetes was Democedes, who was skilled in medicine. Darius ordered that he should be led in as soon as possible. He was brought wearing rags and dragging his fetters. Darius asked him whether he knew medicine, but Democedes was very unwilling to admit it, since he might then be prevented from returning to Greece at all. Darius, however, was informed that the Greek really did have medical knowledge and he ordered whips and goads to be brought forth, whereupon Democedes admitted that he knew a little from having worked under a physician. Then he used on Darius the gentler methods of the Greeks, giving him strong sedatives also so that he should get his sleep. He soon restored him, though the king had given up hope that he would ever again be sound in his feet. Democedes was then in the highest favour with Darius, who presented him with a magnificent house.

Later, when Queen Atossa, daughter of Cyrus, asked him to treat a tumour on her breast that continually spread, he promised to cure her if she would swear to do him a service, adding that this service would be nothing shameful. He asked her to help him reach Greece. Athenaeus says that he promised to return to Persia after the visit. Darius sent him with a following of distinguished Persians to spy out Greek lands in preparation for a Persian attack. He was to return with the party, but he might take rich gifts with him for his father and his family. They travelled by way of Phoenicia to Greece and beyond that to the Greek cities in Italy. At Taras, Aristophilides the king took away the steering paddles of the Persian ships and imprisoned the Persian envoys as spies. Democedes meanwhile made his way to

Croton, where his fellow citizens welcomed him. Aristophilides then released the Persians and restored their ships' gear. The Persians found Democedes with his friends in the *agora* and laid hands on him, but after an argument the stronger party among the Crotoniates refused to give him up. The Persians had to return without him.

Aelian adds that Darius denounced Democedes as a liar and a knave for not returning to Persia as other Greeks in his service had done. Democedes appears to have been the most famous physician of his time – the end of the sixth century and the beginning of the fifth. Herodotus tells the story to illustrate the state of affairs just before the Persian attack on Greece, but does not tell of the later life of Democedes. Iamblichus completes the story by saying that Democedes was driven out of Croton with the aristocratic party of Pythagoreans by the democrats under Theages. He fled to Plataea with some followers. At Croton he had married the daughter of the famous athlete Milo.

Less famous figures of the same period are illustrated in E. Berger, *Das Basler Arztrelief* (Basel, 1970).[543] One is Sambrotides, known only from the inscription on his statue, dated 580/570 BC, which was found on the site of Megara Hyblaca on the east coast of Sicily.[544] His father was Mandrocles, whose name suggests an eastern origin: he probably came westward like Calliphon. A marble disc at Athens shows Aeneus of Cos, who is commemorated with the inscription *Μνῆμα τόδ' Αἰνείου σοφίας ἰατροῦ ἀριστου*, 'This is the monument of Aeneus best of physicians for skill'.[545] *σοφία* here means general proficiency. Aeneus appears seated with his hand raised, but the meaning of the gesture is uncertain. He may be identical with Aeneus, great-uncle of the famous Hippocrates, for the name is uncommon.[546]

But the most remarkable sculpture, which with its background in art provides the main subject of Berger's book, is a funeral relief of a physician seated on a folding chair, his right hand resting on a long staff and his left apparently touching his beard.[547] This feature and others have had to be restored from comparatively slight indications, as has also the figure of a boy, who once stood facing the seated physician in the posture of a servant or acolyte, and carried a bottle-like object hanging on a strap from his left wrist while his right hand held up a plant before the physician's face. The object carried is interpreted as a cupping-glass for bleeding. The physician's name is not carved anywhere on the remaining stone, nor is the original site of the relief known, but the style and the subject suggest some Ionian city on the east coast of the Aegean, or on one of the islands. The quality of the carving and the dignity of the seated figure show the respect in which well-known physicians were held. The relief belongs in the region of the Greek world where the Schools of Cos and Cnidus arose, and is considerably older than any of the Hippocratic writings, though it dates no further back than the lifetime of Democedes.

Our next information on the careers and standing of physicians comes from the Hippocratic Corpus. Though some of the stricter features of the Hippocratic Oath cannot represent what all newcomers undertook when they entered the profession, the system of apprenticeship and the close bonds between members of a school of physicians, whether they were kinsmen or not, are likely to have been general. The wandering life that so many adopted was no doubt partly for the sake of a livelihood, since the number of physicians living in Cos or Cnidus or nearby must have been excessive for local needs, and other regions would need their medical services. But it was surely also to gain experience that individual physicians wandered about the Greek world, learning to know local conditions and local diseases, as the writers of *Epidemics* did in such regions as Thasos and Thessaly, and the writer of *Airs, Waters, Places* also, who set down his conclusions for the use of those who followed in his steps. Experience as a περιοδευτής of this kind would be a practical asset, and successful practice in one or two places would bring renown and a possible appointment as public physician to some city.

The travelling physician in his youth travelled with a master whom he served as an apprentice. It would be in this stage of his career that he would act as nurse, giving the patient professional care and reporting on his state when the physician next saw him. The physician is recommended in *Decorum*, and must have been advised long before that was written, to carry with him not only the usual case of instruments, appliances and prepared drugs and ointments for regular practice, but also a second case of these for use on his journeys. He could certainly rent a house and a workshop for his surgery in as good a neighbourhood as he could afford, but it is doubtful whether for his surgical practice he could carry round with him from place to place the massive wooden apparatus needed for extension and reduction. If he did, he would need a wagon or cart like a travelling tradesman; if he did not, he might hope for fixed apparatus which could be taken over from his predecessor, and should surely have been provided with this if he secured a regular appointment as public physician. These public appointments are best known in later periods, but there is no reason why they should not have had a long history.

Military medicine would provide distinctive experience, as one or two extracts quoted under the heading of surgery from the Hippocratic Corpus amply show, but scarcely a career in Hippocratic times, since no Greek state except Sparta and the Cretan cities maintained a standing army. At Athens there would have been more opportunity for medicine in the navy, but even that was less steadily manned than a modern navy. There were no regular fighting services to which physicians could belong.

The nature of the medical career in the Hippocratic age is revealed to some extent in the traditional life of Hippocrates.[548] This material is distinctly legendary, and some of it is most unlikely to be true of Hippocrates himself, but it would not have been attached to his name if it had not been plausible. For us, particular incidents are credible as told of some physician or other. The different versions are those of Tzetzes the Byzantine in the twelfth century AD, the *Suda*, the lexicon of the tenth, a Latin treatise entitled *Yppocratis genus, vita, dogma*, and finally what purports to be a chapter of Soranus' *Lives of the Physicians* on which Tzetzes at least depended.[549] There are also the pseudo-Hippocratic *Letters* which develop the legend further.[550]

The most trustworthy account seems to be that which has come down under the name of Soranus. Hippocrates was a Coan by birth, the son of Heraclides and Phaenarete, and traced his descent from Heracles and Asclepius. He was trained by his father and later by Herodicus, no doubt the famous trainer criticized in *Epidemics* VI, iii. 18 and by Plato. Some say he was also trained by Gorgias the rhetorician. This detail may have been taken into the tradition because of such sophistical writings of the Corpus as *The Art* and *Breaths*, but it also shows that persuasion and psychological treatment of a sort were reckoned part of therapeutics.[551] Others say that he studied philosophy under Democritus.[552] There are certainly Democritean opinions such as the theory of pangenesis to be found in the Corpus, and such a notion is confirmed by the continual contact between philosophy and medicine throughout antiquity. Hippocrates' powers were at their height in the time of the Peloponnesian War. This again corresponds to the surgical references to wounds found in the Corpus, whether the relevant parts of *Epidemics* and the account in *Head Wounds* were or were not written by the actual Hippocrates.

After this training in medicine and in general culture he left Cos on the death of his parents. One suggested reason was that he set fire to the Record Office at Cos, but more likely was the one he himself is said to have given, namely a wish to see what had been achieved in other places and to educate himself further. He was also said to have been guided by a dream to settle in Thessaly. He was admired throughout Greece for his successful treatments, and received an invitation from Perdiccas, king of Macedonia, who was suspected of having consumption, to take a public appointment there along with Euryphon, who was older. This must be Euryphon the head of the school of Cnidus; the story may be an invention. Hippocrates discovered that Perdiccas was in love with his dead father's concubine Phila, and told her of it, so that in the end he cured Perdiccas. He was then called to Abdera to cure Democritus of madness and also to save the whole city from plague. No doubt these episodes exceed the truth in Hellenistic manner, but none is impossible for the life of a well-known physician.

When plague broke out in Illyria and Paeonia to the north of Greece the kings invited him to come to them, but he sent their envoys back with a refusal after finding out what were the prevailing winds in their countries. He concluded that the plague would reach Athens and took care of the Greek cities and his pupils. This story is further from the truth, for according to Thucydides the plague came from the south.[553] The speculations of meteorological medicine appear here half understood. Hippocrates was also wooed with great promises to come to the court of Artaxerxes of Persia, but declined out of patriotism. This story is a little like that of Democedes, but it is true that the physician Ctesias did serve for years at the Persian court, where he wrote his misleading *Histories*.[554]

Hippocrates died at some great age variously reported at Larissa in Thessaly, near which his grave is still shown. There is great disagreement about his writings, for there is no uniform style in the collection attributed to him; some writings are vigorous, some feeble with age. This uncertainty shows that at least in Roman times and probably earlier the Hippocratic problem existed much as now. Hippocrates left two sons, Thessalus and Draco, and a great number of pupils, the sons being the most illustrious.

This narrative has a certain value as evidence for the medical career as it was in the fifth century BC. The pseudo-Hippocratic *Letters* include a decree of the Council and People of Athens praising Hippocrates for sending his pupils about Greece in the time of the plague, for prescribing treatments for it, for unselfishly publishing medical books which physicians could use for this purpose, and for refusing the Persian offer.[555] In return, Hippocrates was to be initiated at the expense of the government into the Eleusinian mysteries, to be crowned with a wreath of gold after public proclamation, to receive Athenian citizenship and to receive sustenance in the town hall for life. It is a pity that these details cannot be confirmed; they show the beginnings of the legend, but not its origin in reality.

The medical profession continued vigorous during the fourth century, as our account of Diocles and Praxagoras has shown, and also the Hippocratic writings on medical ethics, which are mostly of this period or later. This is also the period to which Plato's remarks apply when he describes two different kinds of medicine, the one practised by physicians (*ἰατροί*) and the other by assistants (*ὑπηρεταί*), who might be called orderlies.[556] Men of the second class, whether free-born or slaves, learn their art under the direction of their masters by observation and practice and not by the study of nature, which free-born doctors follow and in which they instruct their own disciples. This style of medical practice has its likenesses to the theory and practice of the Empirics in later times. The slave patients are usually doctored by slaves. None of these gives or receives any account of the patient's illness; they merely prescribe what seems right from experience, but do this as if they had exact knowledge and with the assurance of an autocrat. The orderly then runs off to another sick servant, and so relieves his master of all attendance on the sick. But the free-born doctor visits and treats free men, studying their ailments from the beginning and according to the course of nature and talking with the patient and his friends, and gives no prescription until he has the patient's consent. He works all the time by persuasion.

This distinction in treatment must have been usual, at least between free men and slaves, but it is of some interest that it never appears in the case-histories of the *Epidemics*, where slaves are among the patients. The career of the master physician must have been furthered by his freedom to converse at length with free patients of influence. Indeed Plato adds in another passage that if any physician of the inferior kind who practise medicine by purely empirical methods without theory (*ἰατρὸς τῶν ταῖς ἐμπειρίαις ἄνευ λόγου τὴν ἰατρικὴν μεταχειριζομένων*) were to find a free-born doctor conversing with a free-born patient in theoretical and philosophical fashion he would roar with laughter, saying that he was not doctoring his patient to make him healthy but schooling him to be a physician.[557] It is likely that such divisions and stratification increased during the fourth century as the profession and career became more elaborate. But the general conditions of practice are not likely to have changed.

One individual figure among the physicians of the fourth century BC is Menecrates of Syracuse, who called himself Zeus. Nothing unusual is said of him in *Anonymus Londinensis* but in Aelian and Athenaeus he is presented as one of the greatest eccentrics of his time.[558] He took the title Zeus to show his power, and corresponded with Philip of Macedon. He claimed in a letter that, as Philip ruled over Macedon, so he ruled over medicine; as

Philip could put healthy men to death when he chose, so he could save the liver of the sick and make healthy men impervious to disease until old age, if they followed his advice. Philip replied to him with the greeting 'ὑγιαίνειν', which on the face of it meant 'may you enjoy good health' but here 'may you come to your senses', and invited him to a banquet, accompanied by his followers. Menecrates habitually attired himself as Zeus in a purple cloak, boots and a golden crown, and carried a sceptre. His followers, who were his cured patients, paraded in the style of attendant gods, and were treated as his slaves because they owed their lives to him. Nicostratus, who had been cured of epilepsy, was attired as Heracles, another, Nicagoras, as Hermes with cloak, herald's wand and wings, another as Apollo, another as Asclepius.

When Menecrates arrived with his attendant gods, his party was set to lie on the middle couch which was raised high and specially adorned. A table was placed before them on which was an altar. First fruits of every crop were put on this. When food was served to the other guests, the servants merely burnt incense and poured libations to Menecrates and his gods. Finally Menecrates and they, overcome with hunger, fled from the banquet amid laughter. Menecrates considered that he had been gravely insulted, but the joke had merely shown that he and his companions were mortal men like others.

This is the oddest career recorded of any ancient physician. It is not likely that Menecrates was a quack as well as a man of insane vanity, or his name would not have been recorded by *Anonymus Londinensis*.

The distinction between the fully experienced and authoritative physician, the equivalent of our qualified physician, and his juniors and subordinates appears about the same date as the career of Menecrates. Thus, in Aeschines' oration *Against Timarchus*, a house where more than one physician practised is called an *iatreion* or surgery and a *synoikia* or joint establishment. Timarchus had installed himself for a fee in the surgery of Euthydicus in the Piraeus somewhat like an intern in a modern hospital, though we have no proof that patients were kept in such places.[559] The head of such a group of physicians is called in Aristotle's *Politics architectonikos*, which has in other contexts the sense of supervisor of craftsmen.[560] Plato in his *Politicus* and Antiphon in his *Tetralogies*, or specimens of speeches for a law court, show that physicians could by incompetence or neglect kill their patients without suffering legal consequences.[561] This left the profession particularly open to the entry of unskilled amateurs. Plato however thinks that a legal licence issued by politicians or other inexpert authorities would be even worse, for physicians earn their status by practising as it is; in the other case they could begin at once without that, on any activity in medicine, simply on democratic principles. The most that a physician could suffer was loss of esteem due to incompetence; he could not fall into professional and legal disgrace imposed by a disciplinary body, for there was none.

The best-known example of such an amateur was Herodicus of Selymbria, who spent many years as a trainer of athletes. In *Epidemics* VI he is said to have killed fever patients by running exercises, many bouts of wrestling and by vapour baths.[562] This is bad because a feverish condition will not agree with wrestling, with walking exercises, with running or with massage: this is to treat illness with illness. The word *πόνος*, however, meant both suffering and exertion. Plato remarks that Herodicus, when trainer, fell ill by mixing gymnastic training with medicine, wore away himself first and most and later many others.[563] Aristotle says that many men are healthy as Herodicus is said to be, but no one would congratulate them on their health because they abstain from all or most human pleasures.[564] Athletic training could always be part of regimen in health, as we saw from the Hippocratic books, but Herodicus evidently confused regimen in health with regimen in sickness. His renown as a trainer made some treat him as a physician, and the lack of medical penalties made it possible for him to kill patients with unsuitable exercise.

It was otherwise in the age which began with Alexander's conquests. Greeks were then spread as settlers or new citizens over great areas of western Asia and in Egypt. Great cities such as Alexandria and Antioch might have been expected to produce new patients as they grew, and the standing armies of Hellenistic kings would have needed medical services of a regular kind. There were certainly lucrative posts for physicians at Hellenistic courts. M. Rostovtzeff in his *Social and Economic History of the Hellenistic World* (Oxford, 1941) provides a mass of information on the medicine of the Hellenistic age which can be no more than outlined here.[565] To pursue the subject through his references, particularly in the inscriptions he mentions, would be to write a separate book. In the older Greek world all cities of any pretensions had at least one public physician of experience and some private practitioners. Famous physicians were borrowed during epidemics and wars, and even for crowded festivals and fairs, from such centres as Cos, and likewise distinguished private physicians. Decrees granting public honours to all these men, residents or temporary visitors, are extant and form the greater part of our evidence. On the analogy of these the decree conferring honours on Hippocrates, quoted above, would have been conceived by later writers, or even invented if it was not historical.

In Greece and further afield the trained physicians travelled constantly and in most of the places where they practised they would not be citizens but resident foreigners. By Hellenistic times the mechanical arts were increasingly developed, as we saw in Chapter 6, where surgical appliances and their makers, the ὀργανικοί, were noticed. The travelling physicians must have depended greatly on these makers of appliances and instruments, as on the professional druggists, whose reputation was generally bad because they were not themselves medically trained.

In Macedonia Antigonus Gonatas employed famous physicians at his court, of whom Diocles evidently wished to become one when he sent his *Letter*, already treated. The Seleucid kings likewise had a body of practitioners at court to attend on themselves and their royal household. This medical service was directed by an ἀρχιατρός. It appears too that all the Hellenistic monarchies tried to create medical services for their capitals and armies, and for the Greek population, who would have been accustomed to public physicians in their original cities, at large. In Egypt there was a chief of physicians (ἐπι τῶν ἰατρῶν), who in one case at least was head of the Museum.[566] Rostovtzeff suggests that a certain Chrysermus, whose inscription gives this evidence, was not chief of the medical service for the countryside as well as for Alexandria but may have been in charge of the medical service for the city only, including the garrison. He supposes that there was a separate service for the countryside with its headquarters in Alexandria, having authority over local doctors, who may have received public or royal pay.[567] Similar arrangements would have existed under the Seleucids in Asia and under the Attalids at Pergamum.

Thus in Hellenistic times there must have been many opportunities for a satisfying career in medical service at the courts or about the country, and for private practice too. There would also have been enlarged opportunities for quacks. The medical members of the Museum at Alexandria were in a specially favoured position, as we saw, for they were encouraged to carry on research, and presided over the most famous medical school in the Hellenistic or later in the Roman world. It is not likely that the native subjects of the Seleucids or Attalids enjoyed the care of Greek physicians.

The increasing mass of knowledge accumulated by the Alexandrians did not produce specialists of the modern kind, who concern themselves with one organ or one system within the body. Nor can any indication be seen that any physician thought of advancing his career by such narrowing of his interests. Surgery, as we saw, was practised among their other activities by the most eminent physicians and, in so far as it became separated in this period from other branches of medicine, declined in skill and in the esteem that it enjoyed. Pharmacology also, in so far as it was a distinct specialism, was likely to become dangerous quackery.

Within the Greek framework of rational medicine there were no hospitals nor permanent clinics of a private kind where eminent physicians could direct the work of teams of subordinates. Administrative power, where it existed in medicine, would have been confined to royal chief physicians having assistants in palaces, and to the remote heads of medical services, who from Alexandria directed local services such as may have existed in the villages of Ptolemaic Egypt. There was nothing like the close hierarchy of modern hospitals. When we look in the Greek framework for equivalent institutions to our hospitals and clinics, the nearest that we can find are the great temples of Asclepius and other healing gods, where patients could instal themselves for years; but these are part of the apparatus of faith-healing, not of clinical medicine. The origins of our own hospitals are not within this tradition, but in the military medicine of Rome and in the charity of the Christian church.

In the Roman period the local service of medicine is likely to have continued as before in the old Greek cities. But the loss of Asiatic territories under the last Seleucids may have reduced the opportunities for Greek physicians in the East until Greek-speaking territories in Asia Minor and Syria were securely in Roman hands. By Flavian times it was again normal for every Greek city to have its public physician. In Egypt the prestige of Alexandria continued to be great, and many medical men passed through its school before taking up employment in various parts of the Roman empire, particularly in Rome. Greek medicine at Rome is thus a special part of our subject, though an outlying one in this aspect. For further information John Scarborough, *Roman Medicine* (London, 1968) may be consulted, especially Chapters 3 and 4.

The first Greek physicians to arrive in Rome were slaves captured in the Roman wars in the East. But by the third century BC free men were beginning to arrive, such as Archagathus from the Peloponnese, whose work was particularly to tend wounds, though later, according to Pliny, his sobriquet '*vulnerarius*' was replaced by '*carnifex*' (executioner).[568] He was accepted as a Roman citizen. Later an edict of Caesar's gave discretion to provincial governors to confer citizenship on physicians, who began by serving the army but soon established themselves in civil life too, not only in Rome but in other large cities.[569]

Asclepiades, who has already been mentioned, arrived in Rome in 91 BC, at the age of forty or a little more, and was famous there for long after his death until the time of Galen. He was not only a distinguished physician and medical scientist, but also a polished man of the world. He softened therapeutic methods from the rougher character which they had acquired in Rome, introducing regimen, baths and exercises in the Greek manner. He flourished at the time when Greek culture of all kinds had its greatest influence at Rome.

Not every well-known Greek physician of this period came to live or spent some time at Rome; yet the capital must have drawn many of them to put a crown on their careers. The best-known example by far of a Greek physician at Rome is Galen, born in AD 130 near Pergamum.[570]

Galen's father originally intended him for a career in the service of the state; but he was persuaded by a dream, supposed to be inspired by Asclepius, to direct him into medicine. After the youth had attended lectures in all kinds of philosophy at Pergamum as part of his preliminary education he decided that no philosophical opinion was well grounded; he preferred mathematics and logic, and he kept his interest in these throughout his life. Nevertheless, it struck him as being far more profitable to study nature, as revealed in medical science. He studied anatomy for four years at Pergamum, and later worked on medicine at Smyrna and at Alexandria, where he remained for five years. When he returned to Pergamum he was appointed physician to the gladiators, which gave him great experience in surgery on severe injuries and wounds, as well as in dressing wounds and in dieting and exercising the gladiators. But an attack on Pergamum by the Galatians put an end to the games for which gladiators were employed.

Galen therefore left for Rome – probably in 161/2, about the time when Marcus Aurelius succeeded Antoninus. At Rome he rented a large house, attended medical meetings in the Temple of Peace, and continued his philosophical studies. When his friend the philosopher Eudemus fell gravely ill Galen was invited to join in treating him with other physicians, Epigenes, Antigenes and Martialis. But he soon quarrelled with them and began a series of bitter controversies. His quick temper, hastiness, excessive confidence and petulant behaviour made him many enemies, both among reputable physicians and among the many quacks who were drawn to Rome. Eudemus warned him that his life was in danger. At this time also the great plague began, which was one of the disasters of the reign. For these reasons Galen returned to Pergamum.

Soon afterwards, however, when Marcus Aurelius was mustering his troops for war on the Danube, Galen was recalled to serve in the imperial headquarters at Aquileia. There the plague struck again, and Galen, not wishing to spend his time in camps, induced Marcus to send him back to Rome to care for his son Commodus, aged eight; this he did until Commodus was fourteen.

During this longer stay, his position and influence were strengthened by his appointment as physician at court. He was consulted on matters of public hygiene such as the maintenance of the Colosseum and other arenas. But most of his time and effort were evidently spent on his voluminous writings. In 192 a conflagration destroyed the Temple of Peace and many libraries and bookshops containing copies of his writings. The quality of life under Commodus also made Rome intolerable for cultivated persons, until he was assassinated in 193. But Galen had probably returned to Pergamum by this date.

His career was brilliant in spite of dangers and difficulties. It is likely that, as no other physician, indeed no other Greek writer, left so large a body of writings, most of which was preserved, so no other Greek physician ever enjoyed such success as Galen during his time in the employment of Marcus Aurelius, an emperor who was himself devoted to Greek philosophy.

APPENDIX

THE CULT OF ASCLEPIUS

No account of Greek medicine in the most inclusive sense is complete without some mention of the cult of Asclepius, which existed throughout all the centuries treated in this book. The relation between the Hippocratic and other phases of rational medicine and the faith-healing that was the main element in the cult was a subtle one. The two traditions of healing seem to continue side by side with comparatively little contact, whether friendly and cooperative or hostile and thwarting. There was no rivalry or controversy such as there has been in more recent times between science and religion. It may be guessed that when physicians of the kind that we may with some reservations call secular refused to treat the incurably sick, they were in effect entrusting them to the unexplained powers of Asclepius, as revealed by his priests and by the dreams and visions that patients or worshippers experienced in his temples and precincts and sometimes elsewhere.

This is not the place to describe every aspect of the cult, since Asclepius was believed to give advice or help in many emergencies which were not medical, though they did affect the patient's state of mind. Here Asclepius was the forerunner of the confessors and psychotherapists of later ages in a deeper sense than the ordinary physician, whose conduct at the bedside is the subject of some Hippocratic and later books. We shall therefore treat only those activities of Asclepius which were directed to the same ends as secular medicine.

In myth and legend Asclepius was Apollo's son, a hero-physician – that is to say a demigod – even before he was struck by Zeus' thunderbolt for raising the dead to life and became after this death a minor divinity. Most scholars regard him as being originally a spirit dwelling beneath the earth who gave helpful dreams and visions to those who slept in grottoes sacred to him, and who was later included among the gods by being made the son of Apollo. From this beginning he became in Roman times one of the greater gods.

His place of birth in legend was Tricca in Thessaly, and his earliest associations were with that part of Greece. Later the cult, complete with stories of the god's childhood, is connected with Arcadia and finally with Epidaurus, where his great mainland sanctuary was located. This change of setting may have resulted from a southward migration of worshippers. The Epidaurians seem at first to have accepted that Asclepius was born at Tricca, but later they claimed that his mother Coronis and her father belonged to Epidaurus. For the various versions of the story the fullest record is in the two volumes by Emma and Ludwig Edelstein, *Asclepius. A Collection and Interpretation of the Testimonies* (2 vols., Baltimore, 1945), the first consisting of interpretation, the second of a mass of texts which provide the evidence for the interpretation. We are not, however, concerned here with myth or legend concerning the remote pre-Classical past, but with the procedure of Asclepius as a divine healer, that is to say, with temple medicine.

It should be noted first that Asclepius' temple on Cos, which became no less famous than its parent foundation at Epidaurus, is now known to have been built and established with its full cult in the fourth century, that is to say in the century following the great age of Hippocratic medicine, and therefore cannot have provided the medical school of Cos either with its notions of medicine or with a supply of patients. Asclepius was never the head of a teaching hospital in Hippocratic times. R. Herzog, the excavator of Cos, asserts this date definitely for the temple on Cos and draws this conclusion in Chapter VI of his study *Die Wunderheilungen von Epidauros* (Leipzig, 1931, pp. 139 ff).

The practice of temple medicine can be studied in two main bodies of evidence, the Epidaurian *Iamata*, records of divine cures engraved on stone and set in the wall of a portico at Epidaurus, and the curious record of Aelius Aristides, the Greek rhetorician of the second century AD who spent seventeen years as a patient and devotee at Pergamum, the third of the three greatest centres of the cult, and wrote his *Hieroi Logoi* or *Sacred Discourses* as testimony to the power and benevolence of Asclepius. Other sources of either kind are by comparison scanty, though they exist. Aristophanes' *Plutus*, on the curing from blindness of the god of Wealth, gives a vivid picture, but much of it is burlesque of temple medicine by an unbeliever.

The Epidaurian cures are a sequence of short narratives of which the more incredible are inserted with no change of style among the more ordinary, so as to gain belief without losing effect. In the present description of them, however, it seems more logical to separate the two kinds.

Among the more ordinary cures, the following may be cited as examples – though even here there is much of the miraculous. The accounts are abbreviated.

Ambrosia of Athens came blind in one eye. After laughing at some of the cures by which the lame and the blind were healed merely by seeing a dream she seemed to see Asclepius standing beside her and saying that he would cure her if she would promise afterwards to dedicate a silver pig as a memorial of her ignorance. Then he cut the diseased eyeball and poured in some drug. When day came she walked out sound.

A voiceless boy came as a suppliant for his voice. After his father had performed the usual sacrifices the temple servant demanded that he should bring within the year the thank-offering promised for the cure. But the boy suddenly said 'I promise'. His father was startled and asked him to repeat it. The boy repeated the words and afterwards became well.

Pandarus, a Thessalian, came to be cured of marks on his forehead. In a dream the god bound the marks with a headband and instructed him to take this off when he left the shrine and to dedicate it. When Pandarus rose and took off the bands, he saw his face free of the marks and dedicated the band. This same Pandarus gave money to Echedorus, another suppliant who came later to be cured of marks. The money was to be offered to Asclepius, but Echedorus did not mention it and even denied to Asclepius in a dream that he had received it. The god then seemed to fasten Pandarus' band about the head of Echedorus. When he took off the band to wash his face Echedorus saw that the marks were no longer on the band, but that his own face had its original marks still on it and those of Pandarus in addition.

Euhippus had had a spear-point fixed in his jaw for six years. As he was sleeping in the temple Asclepius pulled out the spearhead and gave it into his hands. When day came Euhippus departed cured and holding the spearhead in his hands.

Hermodicus of Lampsacus was paralysed. When he slept in the temple the god healed him and ordered him on going out to bring back as large a stone as he could. The man brought the stone, which now lies before the inner shrine.

Nicanor, a lame man, was sitting wide awake when a boy snatched his crutch and ran away. But Nicanor got up, pursued him, and so was cured.

A man had his toe healed by a serpent. He was taken outside by the temple servants with a malignant sore on his toe and set upon a seat. While he slept a snake crawled out of the shrine and licked his toe. The patient woke up and was healed. He said that in a dream he had seen a beautiful youth put a drug on his toe.

These miracles or cures have a certain likeness to those of the New Testament. The punishment of Echedorus is like Elisha's punishment of Gehazi his servant in the Old Testament, who was actually struck with the leprosy of another man because of his greed.

More incredible by far are the miracles performed on pregnant women. Cleo had been pregnant for five years, but after she had slept in the shrine she left the precinct and bore a son who immediately washed himself in the fountain and walked about with his mother. Isthmonica of Pellene first came to the temple because she was childless. Asclepius in a dream said that she might become pregnant with a daughter, but that if she asked for something else he would give her that too. She did not in fact ask for the birth, and after three years of pregnancy came again to ask to be delivered. She gave birth to a girl outside the precinct.

Arata of Lacedaemon suffered from dropsy. She stayed in Lacedaemon, but her mother slept in the temple at Epidaurus on her behalf. The mother dreamed that Asclepius cut off her daughter's head and hung up her body throat downwards to drain. When a huge quantity of fluid had run out, he took the body and fitted the head back on to the neck. When the mother came back to Lacedaemon she found that her daughter had had the same dream and was in good health.

The alleged pregnancies are a medical problem, and so is the advanced state of the first baby after birth. Was it really that mother's child? The dream of Arata is presented as nothing but a dream, and its content is no stranger than that of many dreams recorded by psychotherapists.

Aristides' case is different. The *Hieroi Logoi* which we have are a comparatively small extract, long though they seem, from the contents of a large chest full of notes on dreams, orders and cures which Aristides was ordered by Asclepius to keep and one day to make public for the benefit of the cult. Aristides was a highly educated and intellectual man; but he lived in an age of increasing credulity, and was furthermore hysterical in his own person so that his record and opinions are worth the attention of a psychologist. Some of the *Hieroi Logoi* are included in the Edelsteins' collection, but now the entire four books have been translated by C. A. Behr with introductory chapters under the title *Aelius Aristides and the Sacred Tales* (Amsterdam, 1968). Though much of the material does not refer to medicine proper but to the life and fortunes of Aristides, we cannot linger over that but must attend only to the medical and even clinical activity of Asclepius.

Aristides conceived himself as given over entirely to the service of the god, who decided what his activities and enterprises should be, and in particular what regimen he should follow from hour to hour. This was possible because Aristides did not need to earn his living. After reading the exhaustive rules for exercise and diet, obviously for leisured patients, in the Hippocratic books and in Galen, we are not so surprised at this detailed regulation, which also recalls that of modern hospitals and clinics for certain kinds of case. Long periods of fasting, of regular bathing or again of abstention from any kind of washing, need not surprise us in this mixture of medicinal and religious devotion, but some of the god's other orders, again within the range of clinical medicine, are matter for amazement, and were so regarded by Aristides' contemporaries, medical and lay.

Bathing, whether in the breach or in the observance, was always in Aristides' mind. He was forbidden to bathe for five consecutive years and some months, except in rivers or wells during the winter. Thus in the winter of AD 144 Aristides was ordered by the god to travel to the warm springs near Smyrna, but to use not the warm water, but the river nearby. The river was low enough to be forded and the day was rainy and cold, with the north wind blowing. Again, in the winter AD 145/6 Aristides, who had been lying for a long time too weak to leave his room, was ordered to wash in the river which flows through the city. The river was rising high from the rains and there were to be three baths. Aristides' friends gathered in anxiety to escort him and to see for themselves what would happen. On the way the party was caught in heavy rain, which was the first bath. They went upstream to Hippon to find pure water. On the bank none of Aristides' friends had the heart to encourage him, though the temple warden himself was present and some noble philosophers, for all were in anguish. Aristides cast off his clothes, called upon Asclepius and dived into the middle of the river, where rocks were being churned and timber carried along, and the bed was invisible. But in one place the water was calmer than a crystal stream and Aristides stayed in as long as possible. When he climbed out onto the bank a warmth ran through his whole body, steam rose from him and he was red all over. The party sang the Paean. On the way back there was another shower and that was the third bath.

At Elaea Aristides was sent to wash in the sea. The ship *Asclepius* would be lying at anchor at the mouth of the harbour into which he was to throw himself. Aristides and his friends found the *Asclepius*, and the crew cried out to the god when they saw what was happening. But when Aristides came out of the water the north wind was sharp and he needed covering. On the next day Asclepius ordered another bath, after which Aristides was to stand before the wind and thus cure his body.

These were some of the more spectacular incidents in his usual round of purging, blood-letting and sweating in high fever under piles of blankets.

Enough has been said to show the character of the cult for those who were both patients and devotees in the great temples of Epidaurus, Cos and Pergamum. The large colonnaded buildings, equipped with baths and sometimes with libraries, recall modern hospitals. The discipline to which patients submitted, however eccentric, has again something of the hospital as well as of the religious order about it. Such rigours as those described at length by Aristides were perhaps exceptional, but when patients survived them, as many must have done, they certainly won glory for Asclepius. The patients felt that they were in contact with a divine healing power which might sometimes simulate the methods of human medicine, but did not depend on them for its efficacy. A close study of the drugs and remedies prescribed by Asclepius might show that more of his doings than we suppose were characteristic of the medicine of the day. But these often appear as mere trappings for the healing power which flowed from a science beyond human knowledge. For modern enquirers the main interest of the cult lies in its evidence of psychotherapy performed in unfamiliar circumstances.

NOTES

ABBREVIATIONS

AJP	*American Journal of Philology*
Allbutt, *GMR*	Allbutt, T. C., *Greek Medicine in Rome*, London, 1921
An. Lond.	Jones, W. H. S., ed., *The Medical Writings of Anonymus Londinensis*, Cambridge, 1947
BHM	*Bulletin of the History of Medicine*
CQ	*Classical Quarterly*
CR	*Classical Review*
DK	Diels, H., and Kranz, W., eds., *Die Fragmente der Vorsokratischer*, 6th ed., 3 vols., Berlin, 1951–2
EGP	Burnet, J., *Early Greek Philosophy*, 4th ed., London, 1930
Fuchs	Fuchs, R., 'Anecdota Medica Graeca', *Rheinisches Museum*, 1895, 532–57
JHS	*Journal of Hellenic Studies*
Jones	Jones, W. H. S., and Withington, E. T., eds. and trans., *Hippocrates*, 4 vols., London, 1923–31 (Loeb)
KR	Kirk, G. S., and Raven, J. E., *The Presocratic Philosophers*, Cambridge, 1957
K	Kühn, C. G., ed., *Claudii Galenis Opera Omnia*, 20 vols., Hildesheim, 1965 (reprint)
Littré	Littré, E., ed. and French trans., *Hippocrate. Oeuvres complètes*, 10 vols., Paris, 1839–61
LSJ	Liddell, H. G., and Scott, G. S., *A Greek-English Lexicon*, 9th ed., revised by H. S. Jones
RE	Pauly-Wissowa, *Realencyclopädie der klassischen Altertumswissenschaft*
Rose	Rose, V., ed., *Sorani Gynaeciorum vetus translatio Latina etc*, Leipzig, 1882 (Teubner)
Ruelle	Daremberg, C., and Ruelle, C. E., eds. and French trans., *Oeuvres de Rufus d'Éphèse*, Amsterdam, 1963 (reprint)
Wellmann	Wellmann, M., ed., *Fragmentensammlungen der griechischen Ärzte*, Berlin, 1895
Wellmann, *pneumatische Schule*	Wellmann, M., *Die pneumatische Schule bis auf Archigenes*, Berlin, 1895

CHAPTER I

1 See A. L. Oppenheim, *Ancient Mesopotamia* (Chicago and London, 1964), 288–304, on medical and magical healing and on the character of physicians. Also his article 'Mesopotamian Medicine', *BHM*, 1962, 97–108.

2 On Egyptian medicine see J. B. de C. M. Saunders, *The Transitions from Ancient Egyptian to Greek Medicine* (Lawrence, Kansas, 1963), who notes the contacts likely during the time of the Saite Dynasty (Dyn. XXVI, 663–609 BC). Also editions of the medical papyri such as J. H. Breasted, *The Edwin Smith Surgical Papyrus* (Chicago, 1930) and B. Ebbell, *The Papyrus Ebers* (Oslo, 1939), and *Papyrus Berlin 3038* discussed by Saunders, loc. cit., and J. A. Wilson, 'Medicine in Ancient Egypt', *BHM*, 1962, 114–23.

3 See again Saunders, op. cit., 21–9.

CHAPTER II

4 I, 9 ff.

5 Machaon: II, 732; IV, 193, 200; XI, 506, 512, 517, 598, 613, 651, 833. Podalirius: II, 732; XI, 833.

6 IV, 200–19.

7 XI, 822–32.

8 XI, 514–15.

9 XIX, 455–8.

10 51 ff. Philoctetes, while still weak with the after-effects of his poisoned foot, could yet wield his bow against Paris. Pindar compares him to the sick Hieron. The scholia also describe the treatment.

11 *Posthomerica* IV, 399–400.

12 On XI, 515, scholia Veneti, 453 (Dindorf), and Burney, 87 (Maass), and also Eustathius, *ad loc.*, give the text of Arctinus; see T. W. Allen, *Homeri Opera* (Oxford, 1902, etc.) Tomus V, p. 139.

13 496–7.

14 So W. Schiller, 'Das Hungerödem bei Hesiod', *Janus*, 1921, 37–44, and R. A. McCance, 'The History and Significance of Hunger Oedema', *Studies of Undernutrition* (Wuppertal, 1946–9), 21–2, 28. McCance collects other examples from antiquity and defines the condition generally, offering reasons in the deficiency of sodium in the cellular fluids.

15 45–55.

16 877–86.

17 1072 ff.

18 658–9.

19 E.g. 732–826.

20 *Mad Heracles*, 921–1000; *Bacchae*, 677 ff.

21 III, 64. 2–3.

22 See Chapter 9, pp. 182–4, for fuller details of Democedes.

23 II, 125.

24 II, 47. 3–54. 5.

25 See the discussion in A. W. Gomme, *A Historical Commentary on Thucydides* (Oxford, 1945–56), II, 146–62. J. F. D. Shrewsbury, 'The Plague at Athens', *BHM*, 1950, 1–25, argued that the disease was measles striking a population which had no previous experience of this. The best-known articles on the subject are those of D. L. Page, 'Thucydides' Description of the Great Plague at Athens', *CQ*, 1953, which accepts Shrewsbury's view, and Sir William MacArthur against Page, *CQ*, 1954,

171–4, with a short rejoinder by Page, ibid., 174.

26 For the extant fragments of Alcmaeon, see *DK*, 24 (I, pp. 210–16). *KR*, 232–5 has the most important piece with an English rendering and short commentary. See further J. Burnet, *EGP*, 193–6; M. Wellmann, 'Alkmaion von Kroton', *Archeion*, 1929, 156–69; L. A. Stella, 'L'importanza di Alcmeone', *Reale Accademia dei Lincei*, series VI, vol. 8, fasc. 4 (1947) and G. Vlastos, 'Isonomia', *AJP*, 1953, 337–66.

27 Frag. B 1a on intelligence, from Theophrastus, *On the Senses*, 25. Frag. A 5, from Theophrastus, op. cit., 26, and Frag. A 10 from Chalcidius, *Commentary on the Timaeus* (Latin), p. 279 (Wrobel's text). Frag. A 1c from Plato, *Phaedo*, 96 B.

28 Frag. A 5.

29 Frag. A 18 from Aetius V, 24. 1.

30 Frag. A 10 from Chalcidius, op. cit., 279.

31 Frag. B 2, from Aristotle, *Problems* XVII, 3.916a, 33.

32 For the many extant fragments of Empedocles see *DK*, 31 (I, pp. 276–374) and *KR*, 320–61 for comment. Also Burnet, *EGP*, 197–250.

33 The main source is Frag. B 17 from Simplicius, *Physica*, 157. The comments of Aristotle and others on the cosmogony are collected in Frag. A 37–42: 37 from *Metaphysics* I, 4. 985a 21; 38 from *Physics* VIII, 1.252a 7; 39 from *Metaphysics* I, 4.984b 32; 40 from *Generation and Corruption* II, 6.333b 19; 41 from Philoponus, *On Generation and Corruption*, 19.3; 42 from Aristotle, *The Heavens* III, 2.301a 14; also in 52 from Aetius II, 4.8. See also *KR*, 327–40.

34 The long passage on the clepsydra is given in *DK*, Frag. B 100 from Aristotle, *On Respiration*, 7. 473a 15 ff. For modern comment and explanation see J. U. Powell, 'The Simile of the Clepsydra in Empedocles', *CQ*, 1923, 172–4, D. J. Furley, 'Empedocles and the Clepsydra', *JHS*, 1957, 31–4, N. B. Booth, 'Empedocles' Account of Breathing', *JHS*, 1960, 6–15.

35 Frag. B 105.

36 On the general nature of Empedocles as revealed in this fragment, B 111, from Diogenes Laertius, *Lives of the Philosophers* VIII, 59, see W. H. S. Jones, *Philosophy and Medicine in Ancient Greece* (Baltimore, 1946), 11–13.

37 Frag. A 70 from Diogenes Laertius VIII, 70.

38 For the fragments of Anaxagoras see *DK*, 59, II, pp. 1–44 and *KR*, 362–94 for translation of a selection with comment. For a general interpretation also Burnet, *EGP*, 251–75 and W. Jaeger, *Theology of the Greek Philosophers* (Oxford, 1947), 153–65.

39 The doctrine of matter is again discussed by F. M. Cornford, 'Anaxagoras' Theory of Matter', *CQ*, 1930, 14–30, 85–95, and I. R. Mathewson, 'Aristotle and Anaxagoras', *CQ*, 1958, 68–71.

40 See Frag. A 92, from Theophrastus, *On Sensation*, 27 ff.

41 Frags. A 108, from Censorinus 6, 1, and A 107, from Aristotle, *Generation of Animals* IV, 1. 763b 30.

42 For Diogenes' fragments see *DK*, 64, II, pp. 51–69 and *KR*, 427–45. On his doctrine, see Burnet, *EGP*, 352–8, Jaeger, op. cit., 165–71; also H. Diller, 'Die philosophiegeschichtliche Stellung des Diogenes von Apollonia', *Hermes*, 1941, 359 ff.

43 225–36, 828–30, 930–1.

44 Frag. B 5–7 from Aristotle, *History of Animals* III, 2. 412 a–b.

45 *Nature of Bones* IX (Littré IX,

174–6), *Nature of Man* XI (VI, 58–60), Aristotle, *History of Animals* III, 3. 512b 12–513a.

46 For the fragments of Democritus see *DK*, 68 (II, 81–230) and *KR*, 403–26.

47 Reproduction is described in B 148 from Plutarch, *On Affection for Offspring*, 3, where it is said that the embryo is 'rooted at the navel as an anchorage against heaving and drifting, and as a cable and tendril for the growing and future fruit'. Other passages not quoted in Democritus' own words and sometimes criticized have these points: seed comes from the whole body and its most important parts such as bones, flesh and sinews (A 141 from Aetius V, 3.6); Epicurus and Democritus say that the female produces seed 'from averted testicles' (142 from Aetius V, 1) (this may be the first mention of ovaries: it is likely to have arisen from animal dissection); the sex of the child is determined by the relative strength of the parents' seeds, not by their relative warmth, as Democritus thought (A 143, from Aristotle, *Generation of Animals*); the embryo draws nourishment by vessels acting as roots in the womb, and stays there for nourishment—not, as Democritus says, staying there in order that its parts may be differentiated (A 144 from Aristotle, *Gen. Anim.* II, 4 740a 53). Democritus is here right and Aristotle wrong. The unborn child sucks with its mouth at a form of nipple in the lining of the womb (A 149 from Aristotle, *Gen. Anim.* VII, 746a). It is wrong to say, as Democritus does, that the outer parts of the embryo are formed before the inner (Aristotle, *Gen. Anim.* II, 4 740a).

CHAPTER III

48 See the editions by W. H. S. Jones in *Philosophy and Medicine in Ancient Greece* (*BHM*, Supp. No. 8) which contains a text and translation of *Ancient Medicine* with notes and essays, and by A.-J. Festugière, *Hippocrate, l'Ancienne Médecine* (Paris, 1948). The claims noted are in cc. 1–5.

49 V, 588 ff L; V, 761 K.

50 XIII, 273 and XIV, 676 K. On the history of the Asclepiadae see L. R. Farnell, *The Cults of the Greek States* (5 vols., Oxford, 1896–1909), and Emma and Ludwig Edelstein, *Asclepius* (2 vols., Baltimore, 1945), vol. I being a history of the cult and vol. II a collection of quoted and translated passages. Also K. Kerenyi's *Asklepios, Archetypal Image of the Physician's Existence* (London, 1960), translated from the German original *Der göttliche Arzt, Studien über Asklepios und seine Kultstätten* (Basel, 1947). This subject and these books will be considered again in the Appendix on the cult of Asclepius.

51 On the medical school of southern Italy and Sicily see M. Wellmann, *Fragmente der sikelischen Ärtze Akron Philistion und des Diokles von Karystos* (Berlin, 1901).

52 *On the Method of Healing* I, 1.

53 See Edelstein s.v. Hippokrates in *RE* Supplementband VI, and his article 'The Genuine Works of Hippocrates', *BHM*, 1939, 236–48; also M. Pohlenz, *Hippokrates und die Begründung der wissenschaftlichen Medizin* (Berlin, 1938); K. Deichgräber,

'Die Epidemien und das Corpus Hippocraticum', *Abhandlungen der Preussischen Akademie der Wissenschaften*, 1933, *Phil. Hist. Klasse*, Nr 3 and W. Nestlé, *Hippocratica*, *Hermes*, 1938, 1ff.

54 265A ff.

55 For this view see, e.g. Pohlenz, op. cit., 75–6.

56 For the other view see, in particular, Edelstein, op. cit.

57 *Proem*, 6–8.

58 See the edition with translation, introduction, notes and other matter by W. H. S. Jones in *An. Lond.*

59 See Jones, op. cit., 1–8.

60 *An. Lond.* V–VI (Jones, pp. 34–9); also pp. 19–20 in his Additional Notes.

61 See Jones, op. cit., 10–11.

62 *An. Lond.* VII (Jones, pp. 40–3).

63 Littré VI, 90 ff; II, 12 ff.

64 For this term and a long discussion of the books and doctrines mentioned, see Deichgräber, op. cit.

65 On the Cnidian School see J. Ilberg, 'Die Ärzteschule von Knidos', *Berichte über die Verhandlungen der sächsischen Akademie der Wissenschaften*, 76 (Leipzig, 1924). Also I. M. Lonie, 'The Cnidian Treatises of the Corpus Hippocraticum', *CQ*, 1965, 1–30.

66 *On the Method of Healing* XV, 427 K.

67 *On the Method of Healing* V, 761 K.

68 Mentioned in Galen as author of some books attributed to Hippocrates (VII, 960 K), as skilled in anatomy (XV, 136 K), as author of *Regimen in Health* (XV, 455 K) and of *Cnidian Opinions* (XVII, 886 K), and as writer on remedies (XI, 795 K) including human milk for consumptives (X, 474; XVII, A 888 K). *An. Lond.* IV, 3 (Jones, pp. 32–3).

69 See note 68.

70 E.g. T. L. Meyer-Steineg and K. Sudhoff, *Geschichte der Medizin* (Jena, 1952) 13 ff, and H. Sigerist, *A History of Medicine* II (Oxford, 1961), 290–1, who suggest this hesitantly.

71 Herodicus of Cnidus, *An. Lond.* V, (Jones, p. 33).

72 The other Herodicus is Herodicus of Selymbria mentioned in *An. Lond.* IX. ii, Jones, p. 49 and condemned by Galen (XVII, B 99 K) referring to the complaint in *Epidemics* V, 3. 18 (Littré V, 302); mentioned also by Plato, *Republic* III, 406 A, *Protagoras*, 316 D, *Phaedrus*, 227 D.

73 M. Wellmann, *Die Fragmente der sikelischen Ärzte* (Berlin, 1901).

74 *An. Lond.* XX, 24 (Jones, pp. 80–1).

75 See A. E. Taylor, *A Commentary on Plato's Timaeus* (Oxford, 1928), 504, quoting Plutarch, *Questions at the Banquet* VII, i. 698a ff.

76 See Taylor, loc. cit.

77 W. H. S. Jones, 'Hippocrates and the Corpus Hippocraticum', *Proceedings of the British Academy*, vol. 31, 1945.

78 See note 64.

79 See Ilberg, op. cit. (note 65).

CHAPTER IV

80 After being translated by Dr W. H. S. Jones in the Loeb *Hippocrates* (vol. 1, 12 ff), *Ancient Medicine* has been separately edited by him under the title *Philosophy and Medicine in Ancient Greece* (Baltimore, 1946), with text, translation, notes and essays. There is also the edition of A.–J. Festugière, *Hippocrate. Ancienne Medecine* (Paris, 1948) with translation and similar aids. The full bibliographies given in these editions make further references almost unnecessary here. But it may be noted that G. E. R. Lloyd has discussed the book again in an article 'Who is attacked in *Ancient Medicine*?', *Phronesis*, 1963, where he argues that a principal target is Philolaus the Pythagorean. The book continues to attract attention.

81 cc. 1–12.

82 c. 13.

83 cc. 14–15.

84 This was edited by Dr Theodor Gomperz under the title *Die Apologie der Heilkunst* (Vienna, 1890). It appears in Jones' Loeb *Hippocrates*, vol. II, 185 ff.

85 c. 4 ff.

86 c. 4.

87 c. 6.

88 cc. 7–8.

89 c. 13.

90 *Sacred Disease* appears in vol. II, 138 ff, of Jones' Loeb edition with a short introduction noting its affinity in certain passages with *Airs, Waters, Places*, the text in these being nearly identical. There is now another edition by H. Grensemann under the title 'Die hippokratische Schrift "Über die heilige Krankheit"', *Ars Medica*, Abt. 2, Bd. 1, 1968, with a translation and a long introduction which discusses its subject-matter, its relation to other Hippocratic writings and non-Hippocratic writers in the philosophical tradition, and the text and MSS. *Sacred Disease* has attracted comment from Greek scholars whose interests are outside medicine, from the time of Wilamowitz's paper, 'Die hippokratische Schrift *Περὶ ἱρῆς νούσου*' *Sitzungsberichte der Preussischer Akademie der Wissenschaften*, 1901) onward.

91 c. 2.

92 cc. 2–4; on this part of *Sacred Disease* see E. R. Dodds, *The Greeks and the Irrational* (Berkeley, 1951), 67–8, 77–8; L. Edelstein, 'Greek Medicine, Religion and Magic' in the posthumous collection *Ancient Medicine* (Baltimore, 1967), pp. 205 ff, 215–19.

93 On the resemblances see Wilamowitz, op. cit., Jones' introduction in his Loeb edition, and Grensemann, op. cit., 7–18.

94 See Edelstein, 'The History of Anatomy in Antiquity', *Ancient Medicine*, 247–57.

95 *Places in Man* is best read in Littré VI, 272 ff; on the head and skeleton, see cc. 2 and 6.

96 c. 6, *ab init.*

97 c. 6.

98 c. 6.

99 c. 6.

100 c. 6.

101 c. 7.

102 See Chapter 2, p. 25. This is reported by Aristotle, *History of Animals* III, ii. 512a–512b.10.

103 *Nature of Bones*, 8; *History of Animals* III, ii 511b. See A. L. Peck, Aristotle, *Historia Animalium* (Loeb), vol. I, 165.

104 *Sacred Disease*, c. 6.

105 *Nature of Bones*, 9; *Epidemics* II, 4.1 has the same passage.

106 *Nature of Man*, 11; see also Jones' translation in vol. IV of the Loeb edition.

107 The term *τόνοι* of *Nature of Bones*, 10 is the oldest expression known for nerves in Greek medicine, apart from the *πόροι* which are probably the optic nerves in Alcmaeon but are thought to be hollow.

The τόνοι are strings which have no suggestion of hollowness.
108 This is apparently the same as the primal vessel of *Nature of Bones*, next to be mentioned.
109 *Heart* has been separately edited by F. C. Unger under the title *Liber Hippocraticus* περὶ καρδίης (Leiden, 1923).
110 c. 6.
111 This book gives the fullest account of the anatomy of the skull and of the meninges. The meninges are mentioned in cc. 1, 15 and 21.
112 c. 2.
113 c. 8.
114 c. 71; also *Places in Man*, 2.
115 Alcmaeon 24B4 *DK* (Aetius V, 30.1). *Epidemics* in the later books seems to operate with indefinitely many.
116 cc. 18–19, 24.
117 cc. 8–16.
118 c. 18.
119 cc. 1–6 on winds, 7–9 on waters.
120 See particularly the 'constitutions' in *Epidemics* I, 1–3, 3–12, 13–26 and III, 2–16. The other 'constitutions' are not so well defined.
121 *Humours* has been called the eighth book of *Epidemics* and is grouped with *Epidemics* I–VII by Deichgräber, *Die Epidemien und das Corpus Hippocraticum* (Berlin, 1933), 76 ff.
122 *Nature of Man* has been separately edited by O. Villaret under the title *Hippocrates De Natura Hominis* (1911). It is discussed by Deichgräber, op. cit., 105–12. Its description of the vascular system is attributed by Aristotle, *History of Animals* III, iii. 512b 12 ff, to Polybus, who is known to have been the son-in-law of Hippocrates.
123 For phlegm, see c. 7.
124 For blood, see c. 8.
125 For yellow bile, see c. 15.
126 For black bile, see c. 15 *ad fin.*
127 This four-fold cycle is compared with Empedocles' four 'roots' on substances in the universe.
128 See *Sacred Disease*, 7 ff and 21.
129 ibid., 7.
130 ibid., 19.
131 This has been edited by A. Nelson, *Die hippokratische Schrift* περὶ φυσῶν. *Text und Studien* (Uppsala, 1909).
132 c. 3 *ad fin.*
133 c. 7 *ad fin.*
134 c. 9.
135 c. 8.
136 c. 12.
137 c. 13.
138 c. 14.
139 IV, 36, 40. Cf. *Internal Affections*, 24; dropsy from the liver, 27–9.
140 c. 5.
141 c. 16.
142 c. 4.
143 cc. 1–2. This book is discussed by Deichgräber, *Hippokrates über Entstehung und Aufbau des menschlichen Körpers* (Leipzig and Berlin, 1935).
144 See the chapters on these general problems which make up most of this short book, especially cc. 3 and 4. There is some awareness of embryology, but the growth of the organs is not closely considered within that framework.
145 The opening chapters give this impression to anyone who has read the accounts of the origin of life in the nature philosophers.
146 c. 1.
147 c. 1.
148 *Nature of Women*, cc. 3–9; *Diseases of Women*, cc. 123–53.
149 *Epidemics* II, Section VI, 15; so also *Epidemics* VI, 21, 25; *Prorrhetica*, c. 24.
150 c. 21. So too *Glands*, 16.
151 c. 14.

152 c. 5. *Generation* can now be read in the Budé edition of R. Joly (*Hippocrate*, Tome XI, 1970).
153 cc. 1–2.
154 c. 22.
155 *Generation*, 7.
156 ibid., 8–9.
157 ibid., 12–13.
158 *Nature of Child*, 28. *Nature of Child* has now appeared in Joly's edition (see note 152).
159 ibid., 31.
160 Both now in Joly's edition, loc. cit.
161 Much of it consists of extracts from *Diseases of Women* and *Sterile Women*.
162 On the theory of pangenesis, that is, of direct contribution to the body of the embryo in all its parts from the corresponding parts of the parents' bodies, see Erna Lesky's exhaustive paper on the ancient theories of reproduction, 'Die Zeugungs- und Vererbungslehren der Antike und ihr Nachwirken' (*Abhandlungen der geistes und sozialwissenschaftliche Klasse der Akademie der Wissenschaften in Mainz*, 1950, Nr 19, section D, *Die Pangenesislehre*, 1294–1333). The rest deals with other theories: the earlier one also found in the Hippocratic Corpus, that the seed is formed from the brain and the spinal marrow, and the later one that it is formed from the blood. To an uninformed speculator these various notions would have seemed quite incompatible with one another. The nature of female 'seed' or of the female contribution to the embryo was especially ill-defined until the nature of ovaries began to be understood. The same paper carries the story through the thought of Aristotle, of the Alexandrians, and of the Stoics, with the medical theories that arose from these.
163 II. In this and the following chapters not all the symptoms are reproduced, because the account would be too long.
164 loc. cit.
165 ibid., III.
166 loc. cit.
167 loc. cit., *ad fin.*
168 c. 4.
169 c. 5.
170 c. 6.
171 c. 7.
172 c. 11.
173 c. 12.
174 loc. cit., *ad fin.* Thus is part of an account of empyema, but seems to have a wider application.
175 XV–XVIII, cc. 15–18.
176 XIX, c. 19.
177 c. 23, Jones (Littré I, iii. 10, 668 ff).
178 See W. Jaeger, *Paideia* (Oxford, 1939), III, 19–20.
179 Thasos is the scene of the first *katastasis* at the beginning of *Epidemics* I, also of the second in ch. 4 there, and of the third in ch. 7. It is also presumably the scene of the case-histories, though it is mentioned only in the fourth.
180 *Epidemics* I, case i (Littré II, 684–6).
181 I, case vii (II, 700–2).
182 I, case ix (II, 704).
183 I, case xi (II, 708–10).
184 cc. 6–15 (III, 80–92).
185 c. 13 (III, 92 ff).
186 *Epidemics* I, 1 (II, 596–604).
187 V, 45 (V, 234).
188 V, 46 (V, 234).
189 V, 47 (V, 234).
190 VII, 32 (V, 400–2).
191 VII, 31 (V, 400).
192 VII, 36 (V, 404).
193 V, 95 (V, 254–6).
194 V, 81 (VII, 86).
195 VII, 86 (V, 444).
196 VI, 8. 10 (V, 348).

197 *Diseases* I, cc. 12–16 (Littré V, 160–71). *Diseases* II, cc. 48–9 (VII, 72–6). *Internal Affections:* phthisis, c. 10 (VII, 188–98); nephritis, cc. 14–17 (VII, 202–10); leucophlegmasia, c. 21 (VII, 218–20); dropsy, cc. 22–6 (VII, 220–36); hepatitis, 27–30 (VII, 236–44); diseases of the spleen, cc. 30–4 (VII, 244–52); jaundice, cc. 35–8 (VII, 252–60); tetanus, cc. 52–4 (VII, 298–302).

198 Littré VI, 140 ff.

199 cc. 2–3 (Littré VI, 143–6).

200 R. Fåhraeus, 'Terapiens tre huvudepoker', *Lychnos*, 1943, 33–42.

201 c. 1.

202 c. 2.

203 II, cc. 40–6 (vegetables), 46–54 (meats and fish), 55 (fruits).

204 II, 17 (baths), 58 (oiling, sweat, sexual intercourse), 56 (sleep, waking).

205 II, c. 41.

206 II, cc. 64–6.

207 c. 1.

208 c. 2.

209 c. 3.

210 c. 4.

211 c. 7.

212 c. 2 names the diseases reported in our text; it seems odd that no diseases specifically below the diaphragm are treated as acute. For criticism of the *Cnidian Sentences* see c. 1; on diet (particularly preparations of barley) see cc. 6–10.

213 On the administration of barley-gruel see cc. 4–8.

214 On pain in the side as a contra-indication for gruel see c. 7; also on pains in general as found in acute fever.

215 For the pure juice see c. 6.

216 On oxymel and hydromel see cc. 6 and 15–17.

217 c. 11.

218 c. 11.

219 c. 14.

220 c. 14.

221 c. 15.

222 c. 14.

223 c. 17.

224 c. 18.

225 c. 8.

226 c. 1.

227 c. 5.

228 Section V, i (Littré V, 314).

229 c. 1.

230 c. 87.

231 c. 4.

232 c. 13.

233 Fomentations, c. 21; venesection, 22, in the *Appendix*.

234 cc. 2–3.

235 c. 4.

236 c. 5.

237 *Aphorisms* VI, xxxvi – relief of dysuria; xlvii – bleeding should be done in spring; xlvi – bleeding for pains in the eyes, strangury and dysuria relieved by bleeding the internal veins. *Epidemics* II, 3. 14 mentions venesections that needed to be ligatured; II, 4. 5 speaks oddly of bleeding from the foot of a woman to ease the pain of a displaced womb; II, 5. 1 advises bleeding as part of the treatment of head wounds, if there is no fever; 5. 5 mentions it as a remedy for pneumatosis; 5. 7 recommends it for sudden loss of speech; 5. 10 advises bleeding of inner veins (veins on the inside of the arm), for dropsy; 5. 20 advises bleeding for gangrene; *Epidemics* IV, 61 mentions it for an affection of the testicles accompanied by a cough; *Epidemics* V, 6 advises bleeding of each arm to the point of exhaustion as a relief for a digestive disorder.

238 *Epidemics* V, 7; but bleeding in a similar case was successful for cure (V. 8).

239 This remark is found in many manuscripts and is printed in Littré II, 164 at the end of c. 18, but the

Paris Manuscript 2269 and many editors omit it.

240 c. 27.

241 *Aphorisms*, c. 44; *Epidemics* IV, c. 4; *Coan Prognoses* II, cc. 23, 403.

242 c. 11.

243 c. 44.

244 cc. 17–20.

245 c. 26. So also in abdominal abscess at cc. 29 and 30.

246 *Joints*, c. 40; *Places in Man*, c. 40.

247 c. 47 and Littré's introduction to this book, p. 5.

248 cc. 4, 5.

249 c. 29.

250 *Affections*, cc. 9, 15, 18, 23, 28.

251 cc. 1–3.

252 cc. 4, 11, on vegetable remedies; mullein is *φλόμος*, *Verbascum sinuatum* L (LSJ), rock plant is *ἐπίπετρον*, *Sedum acre* or *album* L (Littré). ibid; hulwort is *πόλιον*, *Teucrum polium* L (LSJ).

253 Horehound is *πράτιον*, *Marrubium vulgare* L (LSJ). (c. 11.)

254 Organy is *ὀρίγανον*, *origanum heracleoticum* L (LSJ). (c. 11.)

255 Houndsberry is *στρύχνος*, *Solanum nigrum* L (LSJ). (c. 11.)

256 Nose-smart is *σαυρίδιον*, apparently a kind of pungent cress, *Lepidum sativum*. All the herbs mentioned in the last few notes would have an astringent effect. (c. 11.)

257 Lithargyrus is lead monoxide (LSJ). Molybdaina is perhaps sulphuret of lead (LSJ). Mineral remedies: c.13.

258 c. 4. There are several other disorders mentioned in this book which have a general likeness: see cc. 6, 12, 13, 19.

259 See cc. 9, 26–7. Littré renders 'angina'.

260 c. 26.

261 *Diseases* III, c. 10.

262 ibid., II, c. 15.

263 Nasal polypus is treated at II, cc. 33–6.

264 cc. 1–7.

265 c. 8.

266 cc. 9–10.

267 cc. 12–29.

268 c. 30.

269 cc. 1–7.

270 c. 8 *ad fin.*

271 c. 26.

272 cc. 27–9.

273 cc. 41–8.

274 cc. 50–60.

275 cc. 70–9.

276 This criticism was made by Ctesias (according to Galen, *Commentary on Joints* IV, 40) and also by Hegetor, one of the Herophileans at Alexandria. See Littré IV, 33–4, in his preface to *Joints.*

277 c. 42. For a recent commentary and discussion with illustrations, see M. Michler, 'Die Klumpfusslehre der Hippokratiken', *Sudhoffs Archiv*, Beiheft 2 (Wiesbaden, 1963).

278 *Joints*, c. 68.

279 c. 2.

280 cc. 4–8.

281 cc. 9–12.

282 cc. 13–17.

283 c. 21.

284 c. 13 *ad fin.*

285 See Jones' Loeb *Hippocrates*, vol. III, 57.

286 cc. 1–3.

287 loc. cit.

288 cc. 3–8. Some phrases in this passage are still disputed.

289 cc. 10–13.

290 I, 62.

291 *Nature of Woman*: c. 3 in connection with displacement of the mouth of the womb; c. 8 in the case of oblique displacement of the womb. cc. 13 and 45 in cases of gaping at the mouth of the womb; c. 16 in cases of metrorrhagia; c. 17 where the womb is excessively moist; cc. 18

and 59 on suppression of menstruation; cc. 23, 71, 74 on absence of menstruation; 33 on emmenagogues. These references and those next to be listed are given to show the close attention of the Cnidian physicians to ordinary gynaecological troubles. They did not neglect these in order to attend only to the more alarming disorders. Indeed the latter could follow if the former were neglected. The Cnidian preoccupation with detail must have brought its rewards here. Gynaecological investigation was also a means of learning much about the interior of the body without surgical incision. *Diseases of Women* I, c. 1: menstruation causes less discomfort in women who have born children; c. 2: result of suppressed menstruation in childless women said to be displacement of womb and disease elsewhere; c. 4: defective quantity of menstruation; c. 5: excessive menstruation, and its results; c. 7: 'bilious' menstruation; c. 9: 'phlegmy' menstruation; c. 74: emmenagogues; c. 86: fumigation as an emmenagogue. *Diseases of Women* II, c. 110: suppressed menstruation said to be the cause of metrorrhagia, also of metritis in c. 127; c. 123: menstruation resumed after cure of chronic displacement of the womb; c. 134: defective menstruation following on hardening of the mouth of the womb; c. 167: excessive menstruation.

292 *Nature of Woman*, c. 9: poor flow of lochia. *Diseases of Women* I, cc. 26–9: effects of bilious state on lochia; c. 37: poor flow of lochia and treatment for it; c. 39: reasons for it, and excessive flow; c. 41: displacement of it to other parts of the body; c. 48: means of making a good flow and hindrances to flow; c. 72: general remarks on lochia; c. 68: remedies to make more flow.

293 Leucorrhoea: *Nature of Woman*, cc. 10 and 15. *Diseases of Women* I, c. 24; II, cc. 116–17, c. 19, c. 119 (recipe for leucorrhoea). *Sterile Women*, c. 23. Metrorrhagia: *Nature of Woman*, c. 16; *Diseases of Women* II, cc. 110, 112, 113, 120, 196.

294 Metritis: *Nature of Woman*, c. 11; *Diseases of Women* II, cc. 120–1, 122, 159, 170, 171.

295 E.g. in *Diseases of Women* I, cc. 63, 66; *Sterile Women* III, cc. 213, 130.

296 Cancer in gynaecology: *Nature of Woman*, c. 21. *Diseases of Women* II, c. 159.

297 Hardening of the cervix: *Nature of Woman*, cc. 36, 37 resulting from death of the foetus; fomentations are mentioned in cc. 139, 7, 36, 57, 58, 60, 62, *Sterile Women*, c. 35. In this book hardening is naturally very important as a cause of sterility.

298 Carneous mole: *Diseases of Women* I, c. 70; II, cc. 110–12, 113, 115. Remedies in c. 178.

299 The whole subject of 'displacement' of the womb and the consequent 'hysteria' is perplexing because there is no obvious boundary between displacements which would be found by modern gynaecology and those which were assumed in the medical theory of this time. A passage in Plato's *Timaeus* (91c) lays down that the womb is an indwelling creature in the female body, desirous of child-bearing, which becomes vexed and ill if it is left too long without fruit. In this state it strays all ways through the body, blocking the passages of the breath so as to prevent respiration and causing all kinds of malady until it is united with the opposite sex. This detail alone is hard enough to understand, since these writers knew the diaphragm. But the condition described by Plato seems to be regarded as a peculiar result of enforced celibacy, while in the Hippocratic writers it seems to be something that can occur at any time provided that the womb is empty. These ideas would be worth closer investigation from a psychological point of view, with comparative material added from anthropology.

300 See note 304 below.

301 On prolapse, see *Nature of Woman*, cc. 4–5 and *Diseases of Women* II, cc. 142–4, 147, 204 (remedies).

302 See note 304 below.

303 To the liver: *Nature of Woman*, c. 3, *Diseases of Women* II, c. 127; to the heart: *Diseases of Women* II, c. 27.

304 To the head: *Diseases of Women*, c. 23; to the leg: *Nature of Woman*, cc. 40, 49; to the buttocks: *Nature of Woman*, cc. 8, 25. General remarks on this supposed mobility occur in *Nature of Woman*, 44, 48 and *Diseases of Women* II, cc. 128, 149–50. The 'displacements' mentioned here are all of the theoretical and imaginary kind; they are not what we should find natural, normally pressure of a pregnant womb in neighbouring organs, though sometimes neighbouring organs are mentioned. *Diseases of Women* II, c. 137 mentions displacements to the groin, pubis, bladder, hypochondria and seat as possibilities between which the physician has to decide, particularly when the patient is of menopausal age. This sort of diagnosis if it was made known to the patient must have added considerably to the anxiety which arose in her from pains actually felt.

305 Fumigation after childbirth: *Diseases of Women* I, c. 54; for ulceration of uterus: ibid., c. 65; as emmenagogue; ibid., c. 86; for drying metrorrhagia: ibid., c. 115; for drying leucorrhoea: c. 119; against consequences of displacement of the womb: *Diseases of Women* II, cc. 128 and 131. Against chronic obliquity of the womb: ibid., cc. 137 and 140–3. It is not always clear whether fumigation was supposed to restore the womb from anatomical displacement, but in one case at least this is so. For prolapse (in cc. 143 and 144) an evil-smelling fumigation was prescribed below and a sweet smelling one at the nostrils, as if to move the displaced womb upward by a disagreeable stimulus below and an attractive one above. This is surely to treat the organ as a living creature on its own, as it is actually called in Plato's *Timaeus*, 91c, quoted above. There are many more examples of fumigation in the gynaecological books.

306 *Diseases of Women* I, c. 74; *Sterile Women*, c. 230.

307 On vapour baths see *Diseases* II, c. 19.

308 *Diseases of Women* I, c. 68. This was done with the patient strapped into her bed by the upper trunk and arms with her legs bent and fastened at the ankles. The bed was lifted high by the head while the patient grasped it and bundles or faggots were fastened under its feet to absorb shock. Each foot of the bed was then taken by one of a team of four men, and the shaking action was carried out by the team working in concert whenever the pains of labour came on. This was less violent than the succussion on a ladder applied to hunchbacks, because there was no shock of hitting hard ground.

309 LSJ translates *μελανθίον* 'black

cummin', and gives the botanical name as *Nigella sativa.* But another and more revealing interpretation was long ago suggested by R. von Grot, 'Über die in der hippokratischen Schriftsammlung enthaltenen pharmakalogischen Kenntnisse' in Kobert's *Historische Studien aus den pharmakalogischen Instituten der kaiserlichen Universität Dorpat* (Halle, 1889–96), 124–7. Von Grot argues that the expression ἐκ τῶν πυρῶν, 'obtained from wheat', which is several times found with it, cannot refer to an ordinary plant, but is much more likely to refer to the well-known fungal parasite ergot, found on various grass-crops used as cereals, and now usually associated with rye. The German term that he uses is 'Mutterkorn', which implies gynaecological and obstetrical use. As a drug it is said to have a sharp effect on unstriped muscle and to be useful in inducing uterine contractions, particularly just after delivery but also at other times when it is desired to clear the uterus.

310 See von Grot, op. cit., 127, who remarks that some of these are strongly diuretic and that some again produce hyperaemia in the pelvic organs. Examples are: fennel, for fumigation in *Nature of Woman*, cc. 8 and 108, to make lochia flow in *Nature of Woman*, c. 32, to bring the womb near in fumigation in *Diseases of Women* II, cc. 133 and 125; elderberry in fumigation to bring out the chorion, in *Nature of Woman*, c. 32, and in wine to cure tumours in the womb, in *Diseases of Women* I, c. 34. There are many more examples of the use of these herbs mentioned in the text, which can be found with the help of Littré's index. Complete lists of passages would overburden this note and those immediately following.

311 See Littré's index for examples.

312 See Littré's index.

313 For uterine or puerperal ulcers thus treated see *Diseases of Women* I, c. 63 on treatment with flower of silver (oxide of lead). These powders are much less common than other remedies. A list of them without references in Greek texts is given by von Grot, op. cit., 128.

314 *Nature of Woman*, c. 98.

315 *Diseases of Women* I, c. 128, II, c. 245.

316 *Diseases of Women* I, c. 25.

317 *Diseases of Women* I, c. 27, cf. *Aphorisms* V, 52: if milk runs out from the breasts of a pregnant woman, it is a sign that the foetus is weak.

318 On bad presentations, see *Diseases of Women* I, 33 and *Superfoetation*, 4; on dead foetus, *Diseases of Women* I, c. 70, and *Superfoetation*, cc. 5 and 7.

319 *Nature of Woman*, c. 32.

320 *Diseases of Women* I, c. 70 and *Excision of the Foetus* (complete and separate book).

321 See note 318.

322 See *Diseases of Women* I, cc. 77–8.

323 *Diseases of Women* I, cc. 1 and 4–6.

324 On the Oath see L. Edelstein, *The Hippocratic Oath. Text Translation and Interpretation*, *BHM*, Supp. No. 1, 1943. He is the originator of the theory that its doctrines are Pythagorean.

325 See W. H. S. Jones in Vol. II of the Loeb Hippocrates, 255–65.

326 c. 1 deals with the behaviour of the physician in the sick-room. For the rest, not included in Jones, see Littré I, 412 ff.

327 See Jones, op. cit., II, 267–301.

328 See Jones, op. cit., I, 305–33.

329 On all these books see also L. Edelstein, 'The Professional Ethics of the Greek physician', *BHM*, 1956, 39–419, reprinted now in the collection *Ancient Medicine*, 319–48.

CHAPTER V

330 On the *Timaeus* generally see Taylor's *Commentary on Plato's Timaeus* (Oxford, 1928) and F. M. Cornford, *Plato's Cosmology* (London, 1937).

331 *An. Lond.* XIV, 19–XVIII, 8 (Jones, pp. 59–71).

332 *An. Lond.* XVIII, 9–49 (Jones, pp. 72–5).

333 *An. Lond.* XX, 18 (Jones, pp. 80–1).

334 *An. Lond.* VIII, 10–35 (Jones, p. 45).

335 *An. Lond.* VIII, 35 ff (Jones, p. 47).

336 *An. Lond.* XI, 43 (Jones, pp. 52–5).

337 *An. Lond.* XII, 8–36 (Jones, pp. 53–5).

338 *An. Lond.* XII, 36–43 (Jones, pp. 54–6).

339 For the fragments of Diocles see Wellmann I, 117 ff. For Diocles in general see Wellmann in *RE* V, 1 s.v. Diokles and W. Jaeger, *Diokles von Karystos* (Berlin, 1938).

340 *Περὶ λίθων* V, 344.40 W.

341 *Codex Parisinus*, (Suppl. gr. 636), ed. R. Fuchs in *Rheinisches Museum* XLVIII, 532 ff. *De Semine*: see Jaeger, op. cit., 187–211 for a full account. So Galen II, 110 K, V, 684 ff K; X, 462 K; XV, 346 K.

342 See Wellmann, 69 ff, Frag. 30 (from Galen II, 117 and 140 K). On bile as causing inflammations and phlegm and causing catarrh see Galen XV, 347; V, 683 K. On external causes of disease, Wellmann, Frag. 31. On the heart and the governing organ and controller of *pneuma*, Fuchs, 5, 543 (Tertullian, *De Anima*, 15). On *pneuma* as carried about the body see Wellmann, Frag. 17. For blocking of *pneuma* as cause of death see Wellmann, *pneumatische Schule*, 140.

343 On blocking of *pneuma* by phlegm in the vessels, see Wellmann, Frags. 40, 43, 51, 63. *Cf. Sacred Disease*, 4.

344 Diseases due to blocking: fever, reduced by breathing, Galen IV, 47 K; by perspiration, Galen XI, 473; visible sweat considered unnatural; Wellmann, Frag. 12. Heart as seat of intelligence, Wellmann, Frag. 14. *πνεῦμα ψυχικόν*: Wellmann, 78. Delirium brought on by phrenitis: Fuchs 1, 540. Heart centre of blood: Fuchs 4, 542; 20, 550. *Arteria* stretching to kidneys and bladder: Fuchs 2, 541; 17, 548. Blood and *pneuma* in all vessels; Fuchs 5, 543.

345 Respiration by pores alternating with windpipe: Wellmann, 82.

346 Digestion, Galen VIII, 186 K; Fuchs 34, 556. Excessive heat causing constipation and leaving undigested food: Fuchs 17, 548. Balance of *pneuma* and food helps digestion: Oribasius III, 17.

347 Bile forces its way into liver through *poroi* (small passages) and so into gall-bladder: Fuchs 30, 554. Kidneys and ureters: Galen II, 30 K. Digestion sharpens the senses: Oribasius III, 171. Seasons and time of life considered in diet: Wellmann, Frag. 84. 141.

348 Male and female seed: Wellmann, Frag. 172. Seed from the branch and marrow: Wellmann,

Frag. 170. Sexual indulgence injurious to the eyes and marrow: Wellmann, Frag. 141. Development of the embryo in twenty-seven days: Wellmann, Frag. 175; *pneumatische Schule*, 152. Boys grow quicker: Wellmann, Frags. 175, 176; Galen IV, 631. Embryo viable in seven months: Wellmann, Frag. 174. Infertility: Wellmann, Frags. 172, 174. Internal teats (κοτυλήδονες). Menstruation: Wellmann, Frags. 14, 60, 171.

349 Signs of coming miscarriage: Wellmann, Frags. 180, 181. Blonde hair and mannish look a sign of fertility: Soranus on *Women's Diseases* I, 9.35 (Rose). Fumigation: Wellmann, Frag. 179. Causes of difficult birth: Wellmann, Frag. 178.

350 On prognosis Diocles wrote his own *Prognostic* (see Caelius Aurelianus, *On Chronic Diseases* IV, 8. 112). Urine a sign: Galen V, 141 ff K. Critical days: Wellmann, Frags. 104, 105. Stages of morbid matter: Wellmann, Frag. 107.

351 For *Directions on Health for Plistarchus* see Athenaeus VII, 316; II, 68; Galen VI, 455 K. Advice against vomiting: Wellmann, Frag. 141, but emetics prescribed sometimes (ibid., 139). Limits for sexual intercourse: Wellmann, Frag. 141.

352 His ideas of fever in heat wounds, inflammation and buboes, of the stopping of pneuma, and of venesection are all noted in Aretaeus, *On Acute Diseases* I, 1. 31. 4. For lethargy see Wellmann, Frags. 44 and 45, forbidding baths and recommending pungent drinks, sternutatories and massage. Epilepsy as due to blocking of psychic *pneuma*, and treatment by bleeding at the outset: Wellmann, Frags. 52–83.

353 On his *Rhizotomikon* see M. Wellmann, 'Das älteste Kräuterbuch der Griechen' in *Festgabe für F. Susemihl* (Leipzig, 1893), 1 ff. *Fire and Air*: see Vindicianus, c. 31. *Anatomy*: Galen II, 282 K. *Digestion*: Fuchs, 14, 547. *Fevers*: Caelius Aurelianus, *De Acutis Morbis* I, 12.28. *Women's Diseases*: *Galen* XVII, 1. 1006 K. *Bandages*: Galen XVIII, 1. 519 K. *Surgery*: Galen XVIII, 2. 629 K. *Prognostic*: Caelius Aurelianus, *On Chronic Diseases*. *Treatments*: Galen VIII, 185 ff K. *Sickness*: Galen VIII, 185 ff K. *Vegetables*: Galen XVIII, 1. 792. *Lethal Drugs*: Athenaeus XV, 681 B. *Archidamus*: Galen XI, 471 ff K.

354 For the *Letter to Antigonus* see Jaeger, op. cit. (note 339), 70–113, text 75–8.

355 For his relation with the Peripatetics see Jaeger, op. cit., chapters 4 and 5; for his interest in their natural science, op. cit., chapter 5.

356 For Praxagoras see K. Bardong s.v. Praxagoras in *RE* XXII, 1735–43 and F. Steckerl, *The Fragments of Praxagoras of Cos and his School* (Leiden, 1958). For his *Physica* see Galen XVII, B 838. 12 and II, 906. 1 K. For his *Anatomy*: Wellmann, 95 ff and Steckerl, op. cit., 47–55. For his views on disease and its signs; Steckerl, op. cit., 70–90; for his ideas of treatment: Steckerl, op. cit., 90–107. Detailed references are all in Steckerl.

357 So Galen XI, 163 K and *Anecdota Parisiensia* I, 395. Empirics said that he trusted too much to creative reason without enough experience, so that he sometimes made brilliant forecasts and sometimes fell into curious errors.

358 For his views on humours, see Steckerl, op. cit., 55–70. He also brought the dietetic theory of Chrysippus and Herodicus to its final form; see Steckerl, op. cit., 67–70.

359 For his physiology see Steckerl, op. cit., 55–67. Galen's criticism: *On the Opinions of Hippocrates and Plato* I, 143 (Müller); see Steckerl, op. cit., 50.

360 For his views on pulses, see Steckerl, op. cit., 61–5.

361 For his notion of bubbles in the veins, see Steckerl, op. cit., 19–36.

362 See Steckerl, loc. cit.

363 On some of these surgical matters, see Steckerl, op. cit., 30–1, 101.

364 On these see Steckerl, op. cit., who includes these fragments on pp. 108–26.

CHAPTER VI

365 Praxagoras' anatomy of the mouth may be an improvement, as set out in a scholium to Homer, *Iliad* X, 325, but his account of the heart as the origin of the nerves, attacked by Galen, *On the Opinions of Hippocrates and Plato* I, 1. 1436 (Müller), was certainly no improvement on Aristotle (see Steckerl, op. cit. (note 356), 49–53). Nor was his account of the two sinuses said to be in the human womb, as reported by Galen, *On the Dissection of the Uterus* II, 905 K.

366 On the Museum as a centre of scientific work see M. Rostovtzeff, *Social and Economic History of the Hellenistic World* (Oxford, 1941), II, 1084–6 and III, 1596, 1598, 1600; also the account of Müller-Graupa s.v. *Μουσεῖον* in *RE* XVI, 801 ff.

367 For Herophilus see Sieveking, s.v. Herophilos in *RE* VIII, 1. 1104–10; also Allbutt, *GMR*, 146–9, Wellmann's remarks in F. Susemihl, *Geschichte der griechischen Litteratur in der Alexandrinerzeit* (Leipzig, 1891), A. Souques, *Étapes de la neurologie dans l'antiquité grecque* (Paris, 1936), 122–4, and F. Solmsen, 'Greek Philosophy and the Discovery of the Nerves', *Museum Helveticum*, 1961, 150–97, especially 184 ff. For Erasistratus see Wellmann s.v. Erasistratos in *RE* VI, 1. 338–52; Susemihl, op. cit., I, 798 ff: Souques, op. cit., 124, 129, 131–9, where he is considered beside Herophilus, and Allbutt, *GMR*, 149–56.

368 See Edelstein, 'The History of Anatomy in Antiquity' in *Ancient Medicine*, 247 ff for the matter of pre-Alexandrian use of dissection as the basis for anatomy. Diocles is treated on p. 257 of Edelstein, op. cit. The passage in Galen is *Anatomy* II, 280 ff K.

369 See Edelstein, op. cit., 248 ff.

370 See Edelstein, op. cit., 253–6, 258–9.

371 On the change of view among philosophers see Edelstein, op. cit., 275–81 from Plato, *Phaedo* and *Laws* onward.

372 Aristotle, *On the Parts of Animals* I, 641A. 19–21.

373 Celsus, *Proem*, 23–7.

374 ibid., 26.

375 Tertullian, *De Anima*, 10. 30.

376 For the controversy on the possibility of human vivisection in antiquity see Edelstein, op. cit., 290–1.

377 *Prognostic*: Galen XVIII, B 15 ff K. *Anatomy*: Galen IV, 596 K; Herophilus as the greatest anatomist of antiquity, Galen I, 109 and XV, 134 K. *Eyes*: Aetius II, 3. 46; Herophilus distinguished five envelopes in the eye. *Midwifery*: Soranus, p. 300 (Rose), mentions his *Μαιωτικόν*. *Pulses*: see references in Galen's many works on the pulse: V, 508; VII, 594; VIII, 498, 556, 592 ff, 645, 717, 747, 786 ff, 853, 911 ff, 959 ff; IX, 279, 453 K. Herophilus was the originator of the pre-occupation with the pulse which runs through much of later Greek medicine and is most exaggerated in Galen. Herophilus regarded pulse-rhythm as a form of music, and based his theory on the musical theory of Aristoxenus; irregularities of rhythm were signs of illness. His *Treatise on Therapy* is mentioned in Galen (XI, 795) and is defended by Galen as based on observation and experience rather than theory (IX, 278 K). *Regimen:* see Sextus Empiricus, *Against the Moral Philosophers* XI, 50 in praise of his *Regimen* for claiming that other goods were worth little if health was absent. *Against Common Opinions*: see the index of authors cited in Rose's edition of Soranus.

378 Galen IV, 596 K.

379 Galen II, 890 K.

380 Galen, loc. cit.

381 Galen II, 570 and III, 335 K. At IV, 646 K Galen remarks on the value of his work on the liver.

382 Galen II, 780 and VIII, 396 K; IV, 646 K.

383 Galen, loc. cit.

384 Galen VIII, 703 K; IV, 171, 731 K; III, 445 K.

385 Galen VIII, 747 K.

386 Galen VII, 605, 702 K.

387 Galen VI, 1. 552. 9 (Müller).

388 Galen V, 543 K.

389 See note 381 above.

390 Rufus, p. 162 (Ruelle).

391 Marcellinus, *On Pulses* (never yet edited), for counting. For differences according to age see Galen XIV, 34 K. Galen defends Herophilus as expert on pulses in his *Distinction of Pulses* IV, 3.

392 For his account of *neura* see Galen VIII, 212 K and Rufus, p. 184 (Ruelle). For his description of the optic nerve, which he called *poros* or channel, a term used as far back as Alcmaeon, see Galen III, 813. Rufus, 153 ff, notes that he identified three membranes of the brain, the four vessels in which the veins of the brain unite (*torcular Herophili* still in modern anatomy) and the network of small arteries (*rete admirabile* in modern anatomy) under the *pia mater*. For his tracing of most nerves to the fourth ventricle of the brain situated in the *cerebellum* see Galen III, 667 K and for the furrowing of the spinal marrow below the *cerebellum*, the *calamus Herophili*, see Galen II, 731 K. There is still some confusion between what Herophilus may have said on this point and what later investigators found between his time and Galen's.

393 Rufus, loc. cit.; Souques, op. cit. (note 367), 124.

394 See Galen VIII, 208 ff (*On Affected Parts*, XIV ff) where he writes of paralysis, with an account of the nerves originating from the spinal marrow and deriving their powers from the brain.

395 The failure of Herophilus to distinguish sensory from motor nerves and thus account for differences in cases of paralysis is asserted by Galen at XIII, 212 K. Yet Herophilus was the first writer to use *neura* regularly for nerves at a time when its normal sense was 'sinews'. The confusion continued because nerves and sinews look rather alike, and because muscles require both tendons and nerves for their movement (see Souques, op. cit., 122).

The motor nerves were none the less called by Herophilus προαιρετικά, conveyers of intention, an expression which recalls our present one 'voluntary muscle'.

396 So Souques, op. cit., 122–3. The notion continued for centuries until the beginning of modern science in the doctrine of 'animal spirits', which Descartes still held. The complete history of *pneuma* is given in G. Verbeke, *L'évolution de la doctrine du pneuma* (Paris and Louvain, 1945).

397 For 'psychic *pneuma*' (πνευμα ψυχικόν) as contrasted with bodily *pneuma*, which supports life but not consciousness and so is called ζωτικὸν πνεῦμα, see Galen XIV, 697 K, as also for the distinction before his time.

398 For 'Hippocrates' as killing live embryos see Tertullian, *De Anima*, 25.

399 See pp. 349–50 of the Greek text of Soranus, *Gynaecology*, in Rose's edition.

400 The list is as given by M. Wellmann, s.v. Erasistratos, col. 350, in *RE*.

401 This Chrysippus the younger is mentioned by Pliny (*NH* XXVIII, 5), Galen (XI, 171 and 151 K) and Diogenes Laertius (VII, 186), who is likely to have transmitted Praxagoras' false theory of *pneuma* in the arteries. He was famous as an anatomist (Galen XV, 136 K).

402 So Galen XV, 306 K on the Erasistrateans. On their attitude to Peripatetic doctrine, see Galen II, 90 ff; Aristotle's teleology in practice withers in their hands.

403 See Galen V, 599 K.

404 Galen III, 538 K.

405 Galen III, 673 K.

406 Galen III, 659 K; II, 708, 716 K.

407 Galen III, 673 K; V, 602 K.

408 For his view of the brain as origin of all nerves see Galen XVIII, A86 K; V, 646. For his earlier view of the *dura mater* as their origin see Galen V, 602, 609 ff K; for his later view, V, 609 ff K.

409 For his remarks on sensory and motor nerves, see Rufus, 184 (Ruelle).

410 The three strands of the nerves are called λόγῳ αἰσθηταὶ, ἀρτηριαί φλέβες and νεῦρα (Galen II, 96 K). For his earlier view of the nerves as hollow and full of psychic *pneuma* see Fuchs, *Rh. Mus.*, XLIX, 550; LVIII, 80; Galen II, 97 K; Rufus, 185 (Ruelle). For his recognition of solid 'marrow' in them, Galen V, 602 K.

411 Galen V, 125 K; Rufus, 184 (Ruelle).

412 Galen: on his ignoring of humours, V, 104, 123, 124 K; VIII, 191 K; XVI, 38 K, especially on black bile; V, 123 K. Apoplexy and paralysis allowed by him to be caused by abundant glutinous and cold humours, Fuchs, 555; hepatitis so explained, Galen XVI, 477 K; jaundice explained by an excess of bile, Galen XIV, 746 K.

413 This formula originated among the Peripatetics with the physical scientist Strato, and was applied by Erasistratus to breathing as the chest was expanded in inspiration and to the flow of blood and *pneuma* through the body. On this see Allbutt, *GMR*, 306 ff and M. Wellmann s.v. Erasistratos, 336–8 and 342–3, in *RE*.

414 Nature as the great artist, τεχνική, is quoted as a conception of Erasistratus too by Galen at II, 73, 88, III, 492 and XI, 158 K, and as provident for all living things (προνοητικὴ των ζωών) at XVII, B 321 K, as fashioner of all parts of the body at II, 81, V, 131 and XI, 158 K. For us the notions of adaptation and function in biology are neutral, implying no conscious purpose, however like they may be to the contrivances of a craftsman; it is likely that Erasistratus himself held a view more like ours than Galen's.

415 This must be so because he believed that the arterial system carried *pneuma* and not blood; but he knew our aorta under the name ἀρτηρία μεγάλη, and many other arteries, for which see Wellmann s.v. Erasistratos, 341, in *RE*, The primal or single vein ἁπλῆ φλέψ (not divided into symmetrical pairs like its ramifications) mentioned in his *Anatomy* by Galen (II, 102, III, 588 K) is the *vena cava*.

416 This is apparently the meaning of διαδόσις at II, 104 K, used there rather than ἀνάδοσις which is also mentioned. Nourishment from the blood is needed for the nerves and arteries that are too small to be visible.

417 Though separate from blood, *pneuma* is assumed by Erasistratus to be required for any output of energy, as in the work of digestion, the beating of the heart and the pulsing of the arteries, and in the functioning of the nerves which are filled with it.

418 For this action of capillaries leading from the veins into the arteries bringing about transfusion of blood see Galen XI, 153; IV, 709, 718, 724; III, 492.

419 For the action of the heart see Galen II, 77 K; IV, 706 ff K; VIII, 315 K; V, 549 K. Erasistratus also knew the valves of the heart; see Galen V, 166, 539 and 548 K.

420 See Galen, *On the Natural Faculties* II, 182 H.

421 Galen II, 120 K.

422 Galen II, 111 K; Galen XV, 247 K.

423 Galen V, 563 K.

424 Fuchs, 554; Galen II, 114 K; V, 123 K.

425 Pseudo-Galen XIV, 746 K. Galen XVI, 447 K; Fuchs, 555.

426 Galen, *On the Natural Faculties* I, 123, 147 K; Macrobius VII, 15. 4.

427 Galen, *On the Natural Faculties* II, 177, 170 K for the veins; for the arteries, Galen III, 537 K.

428 Galen II, 113. 15 K; XVI, 39 K.

429 For addition to tissues see Galen II, 87 and 104 K; for excretion and invisible loss or waste, see *An. Lond.* XXXIII, 40–XXXVI, 25.

430 Cf. *An. Lond.* XIII, 21.

431 On appetites, etc., see *An. Lond.* XXII, 41.

432 On this view of *pneuma* and heat, contrasted with Aristotle's, see Galen IV, 706 K; VII, 614 K; XV, 14 K.

433 On vital and mental *pneuma*, see Galen V, 185 K.

434 Galen III, 540 K; IV, 496, 480, 707 K.

435 Galen III, 540 K.

436 See passages in note 419 and Galen VIII, 714, 716 and 761 K.

437 So it may be concluded from the comparison of the heart to bellows and of the arteries to lifeless channels or pipes in Galen V, 549 K and in V, 167 and VIII, 703 K.

438 See *An. Lond.* XXXIII, 50–1; *cf.* Galen IV, 716 K.

439 See the passages mentioned in note 419.

440 Galen II, 624 K.

441 Galen II, 649 K; IV, 718 K.

442 Portal vein: Galen, *On the Natural Faculties* II, 169 K; hepatic veins; Fuchs, 554, 555.

443 See Galen V, 880; VI, 77 K. Hygiene, an expression first used by Diocles, was intended to keep the body in good order and self-sufficient by avoiding disease.

444 Pseudo-Galen XIV, 692 K;

Dioscorides II, 49. His work *Causes* or *Aetiology* was directed against these Empirics such as Philinus; see Dioscorides, loc. cit.

445 Galen XI, 245, 324 K; X, 377, 379 K. Celsus IV, 31 and Caelius Aurelianus, *Chronic Diseases* V, 2.52 mention that he forbade violent treatment of joints and gout.

446 Galen XI, 148, 176, 229, 234 K from his book *On the Drawing of Blood.*

447 Galen XI, 148 ff K. Caelius Aurelianus, *Chronic Diseases* II, 18. 86.

448 Galen X, 376 ff K.

449 See M. Wellmann in *Hermes*, 1900, 373.

450 Treatment by emetic: Caelius Aurelianus, *Chronic Diseases* II, 1. 54; *Acute Diseases* III, 21, 213; Celsus IV, 18; Galen XI, 180, 238 K. By sweating: Galen XI, 239, 246. By diuretics as in dropsy: Caelius Aurelianus, *Chronic Diseases* III, 8. 146. By steam baths: Oribasius V, 425; Caelius Aurelianus, *Acute Diseases* III, 4. 33; Galen XI, 206, 237 K. By massage: Caelius Aurelianus, *Chronic Diseases* III, 8. 146.

451 Caelius Aurelianus, *Chronic Diseases* V, 10. 127.

452 Caelius Aurelianus, *Chronic Diseases* IV, 4. 65.

453 Caelius Aurelianus, *Chronic Diseases* III, 8. 122; Celsus III, 21; Galen XVIII, A 39 K.

454 Pseudo-Galen XIV, 751 K; Caelius Aurelianus, *Chronic Diseases* II, 1. 13.

455 Caelius Aurelianus, *Chronic Diseases* III, 8. 111.

456 See references in note 489.

457 See Celsus VII, 1–4 on surgery in general: M. Michler, *Das Spezialisierungsproblem und die antike Chirurgie* (Berlin, 1969), 24–5 and *Die hellenistische Chirurgie* (Wiesbaden, 1968–), Teil I, 5 ff.

458 For Philoxenus see Michler, *Die hellenistische Chirurgie*, 58–60, containing fragments and testimonia, and 104–5, where comment is made. The fullest evidence is in Celsus VII, *Proem* 3 where contemporary surgeons are also mentioned. Pseudo-Soranus c. 69 on the cancers (Frag. 17A.1, Michler).

459 See Muscion's translation of Soranus II, 26, p. 106 Rose (Frag. 17A.2, Michler).

460 For Ammonius see Michler, op. cit. (note 458), 136, referring to Celsus VII, 26 (= Frag. 26A).

461 For Apollonius the Mouse see Michler, op. cit., 82 for texts, 119, 121 for comment; for Apollonius the Brute, ibid., 83 for texts, 121 ff, 146 for comment; for Apollonius the Snake, ibid., 82 and 121; for Apollonius the Mechanic (ὀργανικός) ibid., 83, for references, 121 ff.

462 Michler's survey has so far concluded its first volume only.

463 For the Empirics see M. Wellmann s.v. Empirische Schule in *RE* V, 2518–24; K. Deichgräber, *Die griechische Empiriker Schule* (Berlin, 1930), a very full collection of texts including Galen's Ὑποτύπωσις ἐμπειρική (*Outline of Empiric Doctrine*) in its Latin version entitled *Subfiguratio Empirica.* Also the edition by R. Walzer of *Galen on Medical Experience*, the Arabic version with English translation and notes (London, 1944), and L. Edelstein, 'Empiricism and Skepticism in the Teaching of the Greek Empiricist School' in *Ancient Medicine*, 195–203.

464 See Edelstein, loc. cit., 349 ff, 'The Relation of Ancient Philosophy to Medicine'.

465 See Wellmann, op. cit. (note 463), 2517.

466 Pseudo-Galen XIV, 683 K.

467 Galen, *Subfiguratio*, 35. 10;

Celsus I, *Proem* 2, 30; *On Medical Experience*, 87 (Walzer).

468 For the Dogmatist view of medicine see Galen, *On Medical Experience, passim*, and, especially, the dispute between Dogmatists and Empirics.

469 On Pyrrho see Diogenes Laertius, *Lives of the Philosophers*.

470 Already mentioned; Deichgräber publishes a Latin text of the *Subfiguratio* on pp. 42–90 of his *Die griechische Empiriker Schule*, along with an attempt to translate it back into Greek, and critical notes on the text.

471 The Empiric doctrine of the ἀκαταληψία of nature is given in Galen, *Scripta Minora* III, 11.22 ff and *Celsus* I, *Proem* 28. The whole of this description of the Empirics is illuminating (ibid., 27 ff).

472 So again Celsus, ibid., 31.

473 Celsus, ibid., 40–5.

474 ibid., 47.

475 Galen, *Subfiguratio*, 63. 14, 39. 10, 40. 2; *cf.* Galen I, 132 K, Pseudo-Galen XIV, 677, 679 K, Galen, *Scripta Minora* III, 4. This was particularly needed when a new disease appeared which had analogies with a known one (Celsus I, *Proem* 8).

476 See Galen, *Subfiguratio*, 40. 10.

477 For *συνδρομὴ τῶν συμπτωμάτων*, see Galen, *Subfiguratio*, 45. 7; *Scripta Minora* III, 7; XIV, 678, 691 K. For *ὑπομνηστικὰ σημεία*, see Galen I, 126 and 149 K; also Wellmann, op. cit. (note 463), 2519.

CHAPTER VII

478 On Asclepiades see Wellmann s.v. Asklepiades in *RE* II, 2 1032–4 and Cocchi's *Life of Asclepiades* (1762) with Gumpert's *Fragments of Asclepiades* (1794), translated under the title *Asclepiades, his Life and Writings* by R. M. Green (1955).

479 See Allbutt, *GMR*, 176 ff, particularly 187–9.

480 See Allbutt, op. cit., 187–8.

481 See Allbutt, op. cit., 186; Green, op. cit., 125–6 (Gumpert, p. 80), quoting Celsus III, 18 and Caelius Aurelianus, *Chronic Diseases*, 1, 5.

482 This is the view of Democritus, as in Lucretius II, 394 on the cohesion of solid or viscous bodies (*hamatis elementis*).

483 See Green, op. cit., 112 (Gumpert, p. 69), where venesection is treated by Asclepiades.

484 I, 64–105 K. *On Medical Experience* survives in Arabic only, except for a few passages in Greek. Edited and translated by R. Walzer (London, 1944).

485 For Aenesidemus of Cnossus see Allbutt's mention in *GMR*, 164 and von Arnim s.v. in *RE*, I, i 1023 ff. Aenesidemus deliberately revived the tradition of Pyrrho, after whom he named two of his works, *Pyrrhonian Discourses* and *Introductory Outline of Pyrrhonism*.

486 Themison: Deichgräber s.v. in *RE* X (Zweite Reihe), 632–8. On the Methodists in general see Edelstein, 'Methodiker', in *RE* Supplementband VI, 358–73 or the translation of this article as 'The Methodists' in *Ancient Medicine*, 173–91. Celsus: XVIII 31, also Pliny, *NH* XXIX, 6, and Caelius Aurelianus, *Acute Diseases* I, 16; II, 1. 57. Soranus: quoted in Caelius Aurelianus, *Acute Diseases* I, 9. 52. Galen X, 35 and 52 K.

487 See Caelius Aurelianus, *Acute*

Diseases II, 9. 52. Discussion in Allbutt, *GMR*, 194–5.

488 See Allbutt, *GMR*, 197–8; Celsus XXVIII, 28–34.

489 X, 8 K.

490 Thessalus: Diller, s.v. in *RE* (Zweite Reihe) XI, 168–82; also Allbutt, GMR, 199–201.

491 Galen V, 250 K. Sextus Empiricus, *Outline of Pyrrhonism* I, 128. The doctrine of compulsion by the physically universal qualities was called ἀνάγκη παθῶν. *Cf.* Diller, op. cit., 174.

492 See Diller, op. cit., 178, referring to Celsus, *Proem* 55 and Pseudo-Galen XIV, 680.

493 See Kind, s.v. Soranos, in *RE* (Zweite Reihe) V, 1113–30 and Allbutt, *GMR*, 215–23, the most convenient of modern accounts.

494 *Gynaecia Muscionis* in *Sorani Gynaeciorum vetus translatio Latina* (Rose), 1–167.

495 Ἐκ τῶν Σωράνου περὶ γυναικείων, ibid., 171–379.

496 See also the many passages mentioned on p. 1008 in the index of I. E. Drabkin's edition of Caelius Aurelianus (Chicago, 1950).

497 References are found in Rose, 179, 181 and 210.

498 See, e.g., pp. 48, 52–4, 145.

499 On the Pneumatists see Allbutt, *GMR*, ch. X, 'Pneumatism', and ch. XI, 'Some Pneumatist and Eclectic Physicians': also Kudlien s.v. Pneumatische Ärzte, in *RE* Supplementband XI, 1098–108 and the older account of Wellmann, *pneumatische Schule*.

500 On Aretaeus, see Allbutt, *GMR*, 276–9 and Wellmann s.v. Aretaios in *RE* II, i, 669–70.

501 On Archigenes see Allbutt, *GMR*, 279–85 and Wellmann, *pneumatische Schule*.

502 For Agathinus see Allbutt, *GMR*, 271–2 and Wellmann s.v. Agathinos in *RE* I, 1. 745.

503 On the Περὶ πνεύματος in this connection see M. Neustadt, 'Ps Aristoteles περὶ πνεύματος IX und Athenaios von Attaleia', *Hermes*, 1909, 66–9, and W. Jaeger, 'Das Pneuma im Lykeicon', *Hermes*, 1913, 72.

504 See S. Sambursky, *Physics of the Stoics* (London, 1959), chapter 2, 'Pneuma and Force', especially pp. 21–33.

505 On Rufus see Allbutt, *GMR*, 287–9 and Gossen in *RE* (Zweite Reihe) I, 1207–12, an article full of details.

506 V, 105 K. Galen none the less criticizes him strongly, as he did most of his predecessors. Hexameters on herbs: XI, 796 K; cure of melancholia: XIX, 710 K.

CHAPTER VIII

507 Nineteen volumes of C. G. Kühn's Greek text with Latin rendering below, the index excluded.

508 For the life and work of Galen see for instance Allbutt, *GMR*, G. Sarton, *Galen of Pergamon* (Lawrence, Kansas, 1954), 15–24, and R. E. Siegel, *Galen's System of Physiology and Medicine* (1968), 4–18. Also Mewaldt s.v. Galenos in *RE*, cols. 578–81.

509 *Natural Faculties*: II, 1–73 K. See also the Loeb edition of A. J. Brock (1916). *Use of Parts*: III K, entire, in 11 sections.

510 The total of Greek texts is apparently 137. The Arabic and Syriac translations are discussed by Bergsträsser, 'Über die syrischen und arabischen Galenübersetzungen', *Abhandlung für die Kunde des Morgenlandes*, 1925, XVII, 2.

511 See Mewaldt, loc. cit., 589 on *Pseudepigrapha.*

512 I, 56–63 K.

513 See the edition by R. Walzer, *Galen on Medical Experience* (London, 1944), which has an English translation and reproduces also those parts which exist in Greek.

514 On these types of argument see Galen, op. cit., cc. 23–31, most conveniently read in Walzer, op. cit., 132–55.

515 *Use of Parts* III, 83 K; *Timaeus*, 40C.

516 IV, 767–822 K.

517 *Elements*: I, 413–508 K. *Temperaments*: I, 509–694 K.

518 See Brock, Loeb edition, Introduction, and Allbutt, *GMR*, 291 and in *CR*, 1917, pp. 100–3.

519 II, 215–731 K.

520 *Περὶ μήτρας ἀνατομῆς* (II, 887–908 K).

521 *Respiration*: IV, 465–9 K. There is also *On the Use of Respiration* (*Περὶ χρείας ἀναπνοῆς*), IV, 470–511 K. *Muscles*: IV, 367–464 K. There is also *Anatomy of Muscles* (*Περὶ μυῶν ἀνατομῆς*) XVIII, 926–1026 K.

522 *Use of Pulses*: V, 149–80 K. *On Tremor*: VII, 584–642 K. *Pulses for Beginners*: VIII, 453–92 K. *Differences Between Pulses*: VIII, 453–92 K. *Distinguishing Pulses*: VIII, 766–961 K. *Causes of Pulses*: IX, 1–204 K. *Prognosis by Pulses*: IX, 205–430 K. *Synopsis of Pulses*: IX, 550–768 K. Galen had an elaborate theory of the musical rhythm of pulsation.

523 *Theory of Health*: VI, 1–452 K. *Effects of Food*: VI, 455–553 K. *Beneficial and Harmful Humours in Food*: VI, 453–748 K.

524 See Siegel, op. cit. (note 508), 196 ff.

525 See Siegel, op. cit., 241–57.

526 See Siegel, op. cit., 219–20.

527 See Siegel, op. cit., 220.

528 See Siegel, op. cit., 220–1 and 258–321.

529 See Siegel, op. cit., 322–8.

530 See Siegel, op, cit., 352–7.

531 VIII, 1–452 K.

532 X, 1–1021 K.

533 *Unnatural Swellings*: VII, 705–32 K. *Therapeutics*: XI, 1–146 K.

534 XI, 147–86 K; XI, 187–249 K; 252–316 K.

535 XII, 1–378 K; XII, 379–1007 K; XIII, 1–1058 K.

536 *Ὑπόμνημα εἰς τὸ Ἱπποκράτους βιβλίον περὶ ἀγμῶν* (XVIII, 2 318–628 K) and *Ὑπόμνημα εἰς τὸ Ἱπποκράτους βιβλίον περὶ ἄρθρων ἐμβολῆς* (XVIII, 1 300–767 K).

537 On Galen's treatment of amputation see Michler, op. cit. (note 457), 51, where he refers to *Joints*, 69 (Littré IV, 282 ff), to Galen's commentary on *Joints* at VIII, A 718 K, and to Celsus VII, 33 for Hellenistic practice on ligation. Michler also refers to Galen, *Method of Healing* V, 3–4 (X, 313 ff K).

538 See Michler, op. cit., 58–9 on Galen, *Method of Healing* X, 991 ff K.

539 Michler, op. cit., 60–2.

540 Michler, op. cit., 51, referring to Galen's *Commentary on Joints* I, 13 (XVIII, A 339 K).

541 See W. Jaeger, *The Theology of the Early Greek Philosophers* (Oxford, 1947).

CHAPTER IX

542 Herodotos III, 125 and 129–38; *Suda*: see Ada Adler, *Suidae Lexicon* II, p. 42, article 442 (from Hesychius); Athenaeus XII, 522B; Aelian, *Varia*

Historia VII, 217; Iamblichus, *De Vita Pythagorica*, 257.

543 The sub-title of the work is *Studien zum griechischen Grab- und Votivrelief um 500 vor Chr. und zur vorhippokratischen Medizin.* It was published in 1970 in Band I of the *Veröffentlichungen des Antikenmuseums Basel.* It contains also vase-paintings and reliefs, some representing surgical instruments, but its main concern is art rather than medicine.

544 Sambrotides: op. cit., 155 and Fig. 162.

545 Aeneus: op. cit., Figs. 164 and 165.

546 Aeneus, great-uncle of Hippocrates: op. cit., 155–6.

547 See op. cit., frontispiece and Figs. 9–17 and the discussion on pp. 12 ff.

548 On this tradition in general, see Gossen s.v. Hippokrates in *RE* VIII, ii. 1802–3.

549 Tzetzes, *Chiliades* VII, 155 ff; *Suda*: see Adler, op. cit. (note 542), I, 662–3, where entries on the other physicians called Hippocrates also occur. This account is the source for Hippocrates' connections with Herodicus and Gorgias, and it also mentions Larissa in Thessaly as a place that was particularly visited by Hippocrates and where he died. *Yppocratis genus*: in the Brussels MS 1342–50; Soranus (Ἱπποκράτους βίος καὶ γένος κατὰ Σώρανον): see A. Westermann, *Vitarum scriptores Graeci minores* (Brunswick, 1845), 449–52. This Soranus appears not to be the well-known gynaecologist.

550 For the text of these *Letters* see Littré IX, 312 ff. This collection of writings, which also contains decrees by citizen bodies in honour of Hippocrates and lectures and speeches, is evidence for his later renown but not for his actual life.

551 See note 549. On the lack of psychological treatment characteristic of much of the Corpus see P. Lain Entralgo (tr. L. J. Rather and J. M. Sharp), *The Therapy of the Word in Classical Antiquity* (New Haven, 1958). Was Hippocrates himself an exception? (139 ff).

552 See note 549.

553 Thucydides II, 48.

554 See Littré IX, 312 ff. For Ctesias see the summary of his life at the beginning of Jacoby's article s.v. Ktesias in *RE* XI, ii. 2032 ff.

555 Littré IX, 400, 402.

556 *Laws*, 720 A–E.

557 *Laws*, 858 D.

558 *An. Lond.* XIX, 18; Aelian, *Varia Historia* XII, 51; Athenaeus VII, 289 D.

559 *Against Timarchus*, 40.

560 *Politics* III, vi. 8 (1282a3). See LSJ *ad voc.* It may be assumed that the physician Pittalos mentioned in Aristophanes, *Acharnians*, 1030–2 and 1222 was in charge of a group of juniors.

561 *Politicus*, 259A; *Tetralogies* III, 2. 3.

562 *Epidemics* VI, 3. 18.

563 *Republic* III, 408D.

564 *Rhetoric* F 5, 1361 L.

565 Vol. II, 1088–94 in the text; vol. III, 1599–1600 in the notes.

566 Rostovtzeff, op. cit. II, 1091.

567 Rostovtzeff, op. cit. II, 1091–2.

568 *NH* XXIX, vi.

569 Suetonius, *Julius Caesar*, 42.

570 For Galen's career see G. Sarton, *Galen of Pergamon* (Lawrence, Kansas, 1954).

SOURCES OF ILLUSTRATIONS

Deutsches Archäologisches Institut, Rome, 1; the author, 2, 3; Mansell Collection, 4–6; National Museum, Athens, 7; Antikenmuseum, Basel, 8; Trustees of the British Museum, 9, 10; Dr G. B. Pineider, Florence, 11–15

BIBLIOGRAPHY

General Writings on Greek Medicine and Biology

Balss, H., 'Praeformation und Epigenese in der griechischen Philosophie', *Archeion*, 1923, 319–25

'Die Zeugungslehre und Embryologie in der Antike', *Quellen und Studien zur Geschichte der Naturwissenschaften*, 1936, Band 5, Heft 2, 1–81

Bourgey, L., *Observation et expérience chez les médecins de la collection hippocratique*, Paris, 1953

von Brunn, L., 'Hippokrates und die meteorologische Medizin', *Gesnerus*, 1946, Heft 4, 152–73, and 1947, Heft 1, 1–18, Heft 2, 60–82

Castiglioni, A., *A History of Medicine*, revised edition, London, 1947

Deichgräber, K., 'Die Stellung des griechischen Ärztes zur Natur', *Die Antike*, 1939, 16–37

Die griechische Empirikerschule, Berlin, 1965 (reprint)

Diels, H., and Kranz, W., *Die Fragmente der Vorsokratischer*, 3 vols., Berlin, 1951

Edelstein, L., *Ancient Medicine*, Baltimore, 1967 (a posthumous selection of his papers edited by Temkin, O. and C. L., from which the following are relevant here: 'The Relation of Ancient Philosophy to Medicine', 319–65; 'Greek Medicine in Relation to Religion and Magic', 205–46; 'The History of Anatomy in Antiquity', 247–302; 'Empiricism and Skepticism in the Teaching of the Greek Empiric School', 195–204; 'The Distinctive Hellenism of Greek Medicine', 195–204

Fredrich, C., 'Hippokratische Untersuchungen', *Philologische Untersuchungen*, 1899

Fuchs, R., 'Anecdota Medica Graeca', *Rheinisches Museum*, 1895, 532–57

Heidel, W. A., *Hippocratic Medicine: its Spirit and Method*, New York, 1941

The Heroic Age of Ancient Science, Baltimore, 1933

Hommel, H., 'Moderne und hippokratische Vererbungstheorien', *Sudhoffs Archiv*, 1927, 106–22

Joly, R., *Le niveau de la science hippocratique*, Paris, 1966

Jones, W. H. S., *Malaria and Greek History*, Manchester, 1909

'Ancient Documents and Contemporary Life, with Special Reference to Hippocrates, the Hippocratic Corpus, Celsus and Pliny', in Underwood, E., *Science, Medicine and History: Essays in honour of C. Singer*, Oxford, 1953, I, 101–9

Kirk, G. S., and Raven, J. E., *The Presocratic Philosophers*, Cambridge, 1957

Knutzen, G. H., 'Technologie in der hippokratischen Schriften', *Akademie der Wissenschaften*, Mainz, 1963, Heft 4

Küdlien, F., *Der Beginn des medizinischen Denkens bei den Griechen*, Zurich, 1967

Kuhn, J.-H., 'System und Methodenprobleme im Corpus Hippocraticum', *Hermes Einzelschriften*, Heft 11, 1956

Lesky, E., 'Die Zeugungs- und Vererbungsalehre der Antike und ihr Nachwirken', *Abhandlungen der Akademie der Wissenschaften, geisteswissenschaftliche und sozialwissenshaftliche Klasse*, 1950, Nr 19

Lichtenthaeler, C., *La médecine hippocratique*, vol. 1: *Méthode expérimentale et méthode hippocratique*, Lausanne, 1948, and vol. 2: *De l'utilité actuelle d'un retour à Hippocrate. Introduction à l'étude de la médecine hippocratique. De l'étiologie du chaud inné hippocratique. De l'origine sociale de certain concepts scientifiques et philosophiques grecs. Le premier aphorisme d'Hippocrate et ses premisses*, Neuchâtel, 1957

Müri, W., *Der Arzt im Altertum*, Munich, 1962

Plamböck, G., 'Dynamis im Corpus Hippocraticum', *Abhandlungen den Akademie der Wissenschaften*, Mainz, 1964, Nr 2

Senn, G., 'Über Herkunft und stil der Beschreibungen von Experimenten in Corpus Hippocraticum', *Sudhoffs Archiv*, 1929, 290–313

'Nochmals die Experimenten im Corpus Hippocraticum', *Verhandlungen der naturfreundliches Gesellschaft in Basel*, 1929–30, 109–28

Die Entwicklung der biologischen Forschungsmethoden den Antike und ihre grundsätzliche Forderung durch Theophrastos von Eresos, Aarau, 1933

Sigerist, H., *A History of Medicine*, vol. 2: *Early Greek, Hindu and Persian Medicine*, *Oxford*, 1961

SOURCES, EDITIONS AND DISCUSSIONS

ALCMAEON Burnet, J., *Early Greek Philosophy*, 4th ed., London, 1930, 193–6

Wellmann, M., 'Alkmaion von Kroton', *Archeion*, 1929, 156–69

Stella, L. A., 'L'importanza di Alcemeone', *Reale Accademia dei Lincei*, 1947, series VI, vol. viii, fasc. 4

ANONYMUS LONDINENSIS Jones, W. H. S., ed., *The Medical Writings of Anonymus Londinensis*, Cambridge, 1947

ASCLEPIADES Wellmann, M., s.v. in *RE* II, 2. 1632–4

ERASISTRATUS Wellmann, M., s.v. in *RE* VI, 1. 338–52

GALEN Kühn, D. C. G., ed. and Latin trans., *Claudii Galeni Opera Omnia*, 20 vols., Leipzig, 1821–33, reprinted Hildesheim, 1966

The printing of Galen is still in progress in the new Teubner edition and in the *Corpus Medicorum Graecorum*, edited at the Universities of Berlin, Copenhagen and Leipzig

Daremberg, C., ed. and French trans., *Oeuvres anatomiques, physiologiques et médicales de Galien, traduites sur les textes imprimés et manuscrits*, Paris, 1845–6

Helmreich, G., *Γαλήνος περὶ κράσεων*, Leipzig, 1904, reprinted Stuttgart, 1969

Helmreich, G., ed., *De Usu partium libri XVIII*, 2 vols., Leipzig, 1907–9, reprinted Amsterdam, 1968 (Teubner)

May. M.T., trans., *Galen on the Usefulness of the Parts of the Body* (*Περὶ χρείας μορίων*), 2 vols., Ithaca, New York, 1968

Mewaldt, J., s.v. in *RE* VI, 1. 578–91

Marquardt, I., Müller, I., Helmreich, G., eds., *Scripta Minora*, Leipzig, 1881–97, reprinted Amsterdam, 1967 (Teubner)

Singer, C., trans., *Galen on Anatomical Procedures*, Oxford, 1956

Walzer, R., ed. in the Arabic version and trans., *On Medical Experience*, Oxford, 1944

HEROPHILUS Sieveking, s.v. in *RE* VIII, 1. 1104–10

HIPPOCRATICA Jones, W. H. S., and Withington, E. T., eds. and trans., *Hippocrates*, 4 vols., London, 1923–31 (Loeb)

Littré, E., ed. and French trans., *Hippocrates. Oeuvres complètes*, 10 vols., Paris, 1839–61, reprinted Amsterdam, 1961

Kuhlewein, H, ed., *Hippocrates*, 2 vols., Leipzig, 1894–1902 (Teubner: never completed)

Hippocrate, edited by various scholars for the series Les Belles Lettres, Paris, is in course of publication

Deichgräber, K., 'Die Epidemien und das Corpus Hippocraticum', *Abhandlungen der preussischen Akademie der Wissenschaften*, Berlin, 1933

Diller, H., 'Wanderarzt und Aitiologie', *Philologus*, Supplementband XXVI, 1934, 3

Diller, H., 'Die Überlieferung des hippokratischen Schrift *Περὶ ἀέρων ὑδάτων τόπων*, *Philologus*, Supplementband XXIII, 1932, Heft iii

Edelstein, L., 'The Genuine Works of Hippocrates', *Ancient Medicine*, Baltimore, 1967, 133–44

Edelstein, L., ed. and trans., The Hippocratic Oath, *BHM* supplement reprinted in *Ancient Medicine*, 3–63

Edelstein, L., *Περὶ ἀέρων* und Sammlung der hippokratischen Schriften, Berlin, 1931

Festugière, A.-J., ed. and trans., *Hippocrate. L'ancienne médecine, introduction traduction et commentaire*, Paris, 1948

Gomperz, T., *Die Apologie der Heilkunst. Eine griechische Sophistenrede des fünften vorchristlichen Jahrhunderts*, Vienna, 1890

Grensemann, H., *Die hippokratische Schrift über die heilige Krankheit*, Berlin, 1968

Joly, R., *Recherches sur le traité pseudo-hippocratique Du Régime*, Paris, 1960

Jones, W. H. S., *Philosophy and Medicine in Ancient Greece, with an edition of Περὶ ἀρχαίης ἰητρικῆς*, *BHM* supplement, 1946

Lichtenthaeler, C., *La médicine hippocratique*, vol. 4: *Sur l'authenticité, la place véritable et le style du IIIe Epidémique etc*, Geneva and Paris, 1957, and vol. 5: *Les Epidémiques III et I d'Hippocrate, sont ils posterieurs ou anterieurs?*, not yet published

Nelson, A., *Die hippokratische Schrift Περι φυσων, Text und Studien*, Uppsala, 1909

Roscher, W. H., 'Über Alter, Ursprung und Bedeutung der hippokratischen Schrift von der Siebenzahl', *Abhandlungen der königlichen sächsischen Akademie der Wissenschaften* XXVIII, Leipzig, 1911, 5

Unger, F. C., ed., *Liber hippocraticus De Corde, editus cum prolegomenis et commentaria*, Leiden, 1923

Villaret, O., ed., *Hippocrates de Natura Hominis*, 1911

Wellmann, M., Die Schrift *περὶ ἱρῆς νούσου* der Corpus Hippocraticum, *Sudhoffs Archiv* XXII, 1929, 290–312

von Wilamowitz-Moellendorf, U., *Die hippokratische Schrift περὶ ἱρῆς νούσου*, 1911

MEDICAL SCHOOLS Deichgräber, K., *Die griechische Empirikerschule*, Berlin, 1930

Ilberg, J., 'Die Ärzteschule von Knidos', *Berichte über die Verhandlungen der sächsischen Akademie der Wissenschaften, Philosophisch Historische Klasse* LXXVI, 1924, 12

Jaeger, W., *Diokles von Karystos. Die griechische Medizin und die Schule des Aristoteles*, Berlin, 1938

Kudlien, F., s.v. Pneumatische Schule in *RE* Supplementband XI, 1098–18

Lonie, I. M., 'Cnidian Treatises in the Corpus Hippocraticum', *CQ*, 1965, 1–30

Steckerl, F., *The Fragments of Praxagoras and his School*, Leiden, 1948

Wellmann, M., *Die Fragmente der Sikelischen Ärzte Akron Philistion und des Diokles von Karystos*, Berlin, 1901

Wellmann, M., s.v. Empirische Schule in *RE* V, 2518–24

POLYBUS Grensemann, H., *Der Arzt Polybos als Verfasser hippokratischer Schriften*, Wiesbaden, 1968

RUFUS Daremberg, C., and Ruelle, C. E., eds. and French trans., *Oeuvres de Rufus d'Éphèse*, Amsterdam, 1963 (reprint)

Gossen, s.v. Rufus in *RE* (Zweite Reihe) I, 1207–12

SORANUS Rose, V., ed., *Sorani Gynaeciorum vetus translatio Latina, etc.*, Leipzig, 1882 (Teubner)

Kind, s.v. in *RE* (Zweite Reihe) V, 1113–30

THEMISON Deichgräber, K., s.v. in *RE* (Zweite Reihe) X, 1632–8

Deichgräber, K., s.v. in *RE* Supplementband XI, 1098–1108

THESSALUS Diller, H., s.v. in *RE* (Zweite Reihe) XI, 168–82

Special Topics

Allbutt, T. C., *Greek Medicine in Rome*, London, 1921

Baumann, E. D., 'Over de dysenterie in de audheid', Nederlandsche Tijdschrift van Geneeskonde, 1924, 2878–98

'Über die Erkrankungen der Nieren und Harnblase im klassischen Altertum', *Janus*, 1933, 33–47, 68–83, 117–21, 144–52

'Über die Magenkrankheiten in klassischen Altertum', *Janus*, 1924, 241–65

'Über die Erkrankungen der Blutes und der Milz im klassischen Altertum', *Janus*, 1928, 321–37

'De diabete antiquo', *Janus*, 1933, 257–76

'De phthisi antiqua', *Janus*, 1930, 209–25, 253–72

'Die heilige Krankheit', *Janus*, 1925, 377–400

Berger, E., *Das Basler Arztrelief, Studien zur griechischen Grab- und Votivrelief um 500 v. chr. und zur vorhippokratischen Medizin*, Mainz, 1970

Edelstein, E. and L., *Asclepius. A Collection and Interpretation of the Testimonies*, 2 vols., Baltimore, 1945

Flashar, H., *Melancholie und Melancholiker in den medizinischen Theorien der Antike*, Berlin, 1966

Gask, G. E., and Todd, J., 'The Origin of Hospitals' in Underwood, E., *Science, Medicine and History*, Oxford, 1953, I, 122–9

von Grot, R., 'Über die in der hippokratischen Schriftensammlung enthaltenen pharmakalogischen Kenntnisse' in Kobert's *Historische studien aus dem pharmakologischen Institut der Universität Dorpat*, Halle, 1889–96, reprinted Leipzig, 1968

Kerenyi, C., *Asklepios, Archetypal Image of the Physician's Existence*, London, 1960

Klibansky, R., Panofsky, E., and Saxl, F., *Saturn and Melancholy*, London, 1961

MacArthur, W., 'The Athenian Plague. A Medical Note', *CQ*, 1954, 171–4

Meinecke, B., 'Consumption in Classical Antiquity', *Annals of Medical History*, 1927, 379–402

Michler, M., *Das Spezialisierungsproblem und die antike Chirurgie*, Berlin, 1969

Die hellenistische Chirurgie, Teil 1: *Die alexandrinischen Chirurgen*, Wiesbaden, 1968

'Die Klumpfusslehre der Hippokratiken', *Sudhoffs Archiv* 1963, Beiheft 2

Nestlé, W., 'Hippocratica', *Hermes*, 1938, 1–38

Page, D. L., 'Thucydides' Description of the Great Plague at Athens', *CQ*, 1953, 97–119

'The Plague: A Lay Commentary on a Medical Note', *CQ*, 1954, 174

Regenbogen, R., 'Eine Forschungsmethode antiker Naturwissenschaft', *Quellen und Studien zur Geschichte der Mathematik*, 1929, Abteilung B, Band I, 131–82

Rostovtzeff, M., *Social and Economic History of the Hellenistic World*, Oxford, 1941

Schmidt, s.v. Drogen in *RE* Supplementband V, 172–82

Shrewsbury, J. F. D., 'The Plague at Athens', *BHM*, 1950, 1–25

Temkin, O., *The Falling Sickness: A History of Epilepsy from the Greeks to the Beginnings of Modern Neurology*, Baltimore, 1945

INDICES

PROPER NAMES

EXTANT WRITINGS

Lost writings are mentioned with their author's names in the text and are not included here. No author's name is given here for books of the Hippocratic Corpus.

SELECTED MEDICAL TOPICS